Psychopharmacology Series 9

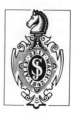

The Hamilton Scales

Editors

Per Bech   Alec Coppen

With 4 Figures

Springer-Verlag
Berlin Heidelberg New York
London Paris Tokyo
Hong Kong Barcelona

PER BECH M.D., Ph.D.
Head of Psychiatric Department, Frederiksborg General Hospital,
3400 Hillerød, Denmark

Dr. ALEC COPPEN
Director, MRC Neuropsychiatry Research Laboratory,
West Park Hospital, Epsom, Surrey KT19 8PB, United Kingdom

Cover illustration:
The three clinical components of the Hamilton Depression Scale

Vols. 1 and 2 of this series appeared under the title „Psychopharmacology Supplementum"

ISBN 3-540-52095-3 Springer-Verlag Berlin Heidelberg New York
ISBN 0-387-52095-3 Springer-Verlag New York Berlin Heidelberg

© Springer-Verlag Berlin Heidelberg 1990
Printed in Germany

Typesetting: International Typesetters Inc., Makati, Philippines
2125/3130(3011)-543210 − Printed on acid-free paper

00807

This book is due for return on or before the last date shown below.

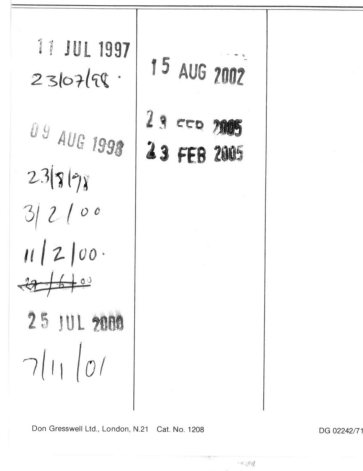

11 JUL 1997

23/07/98 ·

09 AUG 1998

23/8/9?

3/2/00

11/2/00 ·

~~29/6/00~~

25 JUL 2000

7/11/01

15 AUG 2002

2 9 FEB 2005

23 FEB 2005

Preface

The European College of Neuropsychopharmacology (ECNP) is a scientific and educational association which represents a variety of disciplines. The first ECNP congress took place in Copenhagen, May 1985, where a working group of European scientists within the field of psychopharmacology was elected to prepare a constituent ECNP congress in Brussels, 1987. Among the most active members of this group was Max Hamilton. At the second ECNP congress in Brussels Max Hamilton was elected as the first honorary member of the ECNP.

When we received the message of his death we decided at once to arrange a Max Hamilton memorial symposium at the third ECNP congress, May 1989, in Gothenburg, Sweden.

This monograph contains the proceedings of the Max Hamilton symposium which was chaired by the editors. The opening lecture of the third ECNP congress was a Max Hamilton lecture: "A life devoted to science in psychiatry" which was presented by Sir Martin Roth. It seemed obvious to include Sir Martin's lecture as the opening article of this monograph. Although G.E. Berrios was unable to participate in the ECNP congress we have found it logical to include his manuscript on "The Hamilton Depression Scale and the Numerical Description of the Symptoms of Depression" as another personal contribution to Max Hamilton and his rating scales.

The participants in the Max Hamilton symposium have all covered important aspects of the scales constructed by Max Hamilton three decades ago. At the symposium it was found that the presentations followed each other in a meaningful way. The different European and American experiences with the Hamilton scales emphasized their international utility, comparable to the standard classification systems of clinical psychiatry, such as the ICD or DSM. For the purpose of drawing conclusions across studies in depression or anxiety the Hamilton scales are mandatory.

Psychometrically, it seems natural to compare the work of Max Hamilton on affective disorders with the work of Alfred Binet on mental retardation. It is our hope that with this monograph the ECNP has both honoured Max Hamilton personally and paid tribute to his great contribution to psychiatry.

This publication was made possible by the sponsorship of Duphar and the support of Novo-Nordisk.

Copenhagen, Epsom   PER BECH · ALEC COPPEN

Contents

List of Contributors

You will find the addresses at the beginning of the respective contribution

Bech, P. 72
Berrios, G.E. 80
Bulbena-Villarasa, A. 80
Cassano, G.B. 20
Conti, L. 20
Gastpar, M. 10
Gilsdorf, U. 10
Griez, E. 28

Hooijer, C. 28
Maier, W. 64
Mennen, M.F.G. 28
Paykel, E.S. 40
Pull, C.B. 35
Roth, M. 1
Williams, J.B.W. 48
Zitman, F.G. 28

Max Hamilton: A Life Devoted to Psychiatric Science

M. ROTH[1]

The death of Max Hamilton on 16 August 1988 has deprived psychiatry in Great Britain and the world of one of its most vigorous, incisive and independent minds, and a personality of rare boldness and integrity. He had gained worldwide renown for his studies of psychopathology and his contributions to its quantitative assessment using reliable and valid techniques.

Like many men endowed with originality, Max Hamilton's sociocultural origins were complex and probably responsible in part for the detachment, objectivity and the abhorrence of received wisdom that characterised his outlook. He was born in Frankfurt-am-Main in Germany and came to England with his parents in 1914, when he was 2 1/2 years old. He was inclined to attribute his mathematical talents to the inspired teaching of the headmaster of the famous Grammar School, The Central Foundation School in London, where he received his secondary education. He was disinclined, erroneously I believe, to give credit to his natural many-sided talents.

Max Hamilton had stated that he chose medicine as a profession because of the scientific interest of the problems it posed rather than the desire to engage in clinical practice as a doctor. Not surprisingly he was bored by the didactic teaching and dogmatic interpretation of clinical evidence that often predominated in the clinical education a half century ago. "Make the diagnosis while you are taking the history and then confirm it by your physical examination –" was a favourite exhortation of one of my own teachers almost 50 years ago. There was little, if any, heed given to refutation or self-immolation on the altar of truth, in the sense of Popper. Max Hamilton's undergraduate career was therefore undistinguished and, as with many medical men destined to make their mark in science, examinations in clinical medicine were to prove a recurring problem. But once he had qualified, he went on to become a perceptive, skilful as well as compassionate doctor. He continued until the end of his distinguished career to teach students that the care of patients had to be given the same top priority in academic departments within a clinical school as in the course of ordinary clinical practice in the hospital or community. The identity he came to assume as clinical professor was shaped, to some extent, by long-established unwritten law which continues to prevail in British schools of medicine. This

[1] University of Cambridge Clinical School, Addenbrooke's Hospital (Level 5), Hills Road, Cambridge CB2 2QQ, UK

The Hamilton Scales
Editors: Per Bech and Alec Coppen
(Psychopharmacology Series 9)
© Springer-Verlag Berlin Heidelberg 1990

ordains that any professor or lecturer who attempts as far as he can to delegate his clinical responsibilities and never responds personally to requests for consultation should be invisible; it seeks further to ensure that on committees in which he competes for space facilities and funds, his pleas will impinge upon deaf ears. However, the priority Max Hamilton gave to the care of patients stemmed mainly from deep conviction.

1 Early Career in Psychiatry

His career and outlook were characterised by other features that were highly distinctive. A profound scepticism respecting accepted teaching about clinical practice or theory was a firmly ingrained trait. Whether in the most lowly or the highest positions that he held in psychiatry, he probed the phenomena he encountered with challenging questions that called for investigation. Engaged as a general practitioner to aged pensioners and unemployed in 1936, he was puzzled by the recurrent attacks of hypoglycaemia experienced by many of his patients. As it turned out, the scientifically estimated diets they had been prescribed had proved too costly and complicated for this poverty-stricken and deprived clientele.

At the outbreak of war Max Hamilton joined the RAF. He was appointed Medical Officer of a unit comprised of many men who had been promoted or down-graded from fighting units following emotional breakdown. In the hope of discouraging others, the diagnosis that had been promulgated for such persons – who had in many cases flown on 30-40 bombing raids – used the humiliating label "lowered moral fibre". This was Max Hamilton's first close encounter with mental suffering.

Having decided on a career in psychiatry, he took the unusual course of preparing for the first part of the Diploma in Psychological Medicine (DPM), then the standard qualification, without having had any clinical experience in psychiatry. In the course of his readings in basic neurobiological sciences he read Woodworth's "Introduction to Psychology". His was a prepared mind and he clearly understood, for the first time, the difference between the posing and critical testing of hypotheses and other forms of mental reasoning.

2 The Maudsley and University College London and Springfield Hospital

After acquiring his DPM, Max Hamilton managed to gain admission in 1945 to the "Holy of Holies" of British psychiatry, the Maudsley Hospital, where he did not prove a success. A special form of interrogation from on high by some of the "high priests in the temple" helped to make psychiatrists of some, but was not formative for others. Max had a certain respect for book learning but his approach to problems was empirical. He could not conjure up respect for authority, asked too many questions and would accept neither a dogmatic "yes" or a "no" for an answer. Thus, he gravitated towards the Department of Psychology where he developed his knowledge of multivariate statistics and became one of the first psychiatrists to apply factor analysis and later other multivariate methods to psychiatric problems. Although familiar with Moore's attempt at validation of existing psychiatric taxonomy with the aid of factor analysis, the problems Max Hamilton was to tackle were of a different complexion.

A junior post as part-time lecturer at University College, London between 1945 and 1947 afforded a portal of entry to the department of Cyril Burt, whose teaching made a lasting imprint, as did the discussions with the many eager young men aspiring to research careers who had, at that time, gathered around Burt from every part of the world. The later revelations which testified to Burt's scientific dishonesty in certain of his enquiries were to cause Max perplexity for the rest of his life. It appeared out of character and without purpose in a man of immense intellectual powers and scientific achievement. But these revelations were to burst upon the world decades later.

A reasoned, objective and methodologically stringent approach to the study of mental life were to become the main weapons in Max Hamilton's intellectual armoury after his exposure to investigative psychology in Burt's department. Some decades later he was to be elected president of the British Psychological Association, the only clinical psychiatrist on whom this honour has been conferred to my knowledge. From this period there came his lucid and illuminating book on *Psychosomatics,* published in 1955. Its inspiration had issued from investigations into the personality of patients with gastric and duodenal ulcer which had also formed the subject of his doctoral thesis.

After a short period in Kings College Hospital (1951-1952), he moved to the lowly position of Senior Hospital Medical Officer at Springfield Hospital for a 2-year period. He had by then entered his forties. He cannot have been unaware of his true intellectual stature. A lesser man might have acknowledged defeat and lapsed in bitterness and resentment into a state of apathy and inertia. Max dedicated himself instead to the care of the deteriorated, demoralised and apathetic patients treated mainly with sedatives and occasionally with unmodified ECT. He kept painstaking records with a card for each patient, which he always carried with him. A sphygmomanometer and opthalmoscope not previously seen at this hospital made their appearance there. He continued to pose questions when relaxants came on the scene. He discovered a means of checking whether or not a patient had had a convulsion by occluding the circulation to one arm before the relaxant was injected into the other.

A comparison of the results of insulin coma therapy in schizophrenic patients and ECT given to those who had been rejected for this treatment brought to light no differences in outcome between the two treatments even when confounding variables had been eliminated. This report gained the Regional Research Prize but, like a number of other investigations he had carried out, this study was not deemed by him to be worthy of publication. Patients had not been randomly allocated to the two treatments.

3 The Anxiety and Depression Rating Scales

The Hamilton Anxiety Rating Scale (HAM-A) had been prepared for use in a trial of the anxiolytic "meprobamate" undertaken at the behest of Professor McCalman then the head of department in Leeds where Max Hamilton had been appointed lecturer in 1953. His evaluation of the two treatments was undertaken with the aid of a two-way factorial design with unequal numbers in the cells, a model which was to be subsequently emulated in many trials of psychotropic drugs. Placebo was administered for 2 weeks and assessment was made of the patients who had been randomised in the second to the fifth week. The progressive improvement of patients on placebo led to the suggestion that trials of anxiolytics ought to commence with 4 weeks on placebo. This device was to be reformulated afresh some 20 years later by other investigators.

In 1957, having failed in his attempts to secure relief from the heavy burden of clinical and routine teaching duties, Max took a step that required courage and singleness of purpose. Heedless of damage to his chances of academic promotion, he resigned his Senior Lectureship to take up a 3-year research post. The Senior Lectureship was the usual springboard for promotion to a Chair – that is, when it was not used as a sofa on which to recline.

Working at a local mental hospital with which he had always maintained close contacts, he undertook a factor analysis of patients with depression. From the results, he developed the Hamilton Depression Rating Scale (HAM-D), which he submitted to careful testing before its publication in 1960. He was always to regard it as superior to the Hamilton anxiety scale. A large body of additional data derived from principle components analyses of 152 male and 120 female patients with depressive illness was published in his paper of 1967. This contained detailed instructions for the administration of the rating scale. The definition of the terms reflected a wealth of clinical experience and fine discrimination. The rating scale was developed from the first general factor.

Max Hamilton's instructions for use of his depression scale are rarely followed at the present time. Neither the important differences between men and women, nor the clinical profiles defined by components 2 to 5 in the 1967 analysis in particular have received adequate attention or been submitted to the further exploration they deserve.

The conciseness of the depression scale was deliberate. Max considered that scales should confine themselves to the most salient and consistent clinically observable items to ensure as far as possible that signals would not be obscured by noise. Nonetheless, some limitations have become evident in the three decades since publication of the HAM-D scale in 1960. It does not comprise a homogeneous list of items; for reasons that are clear from examination of the original factor loadings. The high loadings of the anxiety items are responsible for the high correlation of the HAM-D scale (0.5 to 0.6) with the (HAM-A) scale. It tends also to be forgotten that it is not a diagnostic but a severity scale. But some workers have used it with the aid of a threshhold limit as a basis for or an adjunct to decision making regarding the clinical diagnosis.

The HAM-D scale was intended for use with all forms of depression. However, although the distinction between endogenous and nonendogenous or neurotic forms of depression has been disputed in the past, in recent years there has been increasing evidence that the endogenous form of illness is a distinct psychiatric disorder; both DSM-III-R and ICD-10 have conceded the separateness of endogenous or "melancholic" states. They probably have a close kinship with bipolar disorder in the light of much recent evidence.

Furthermore, since the Hamilton scale is a severity scale and neurotic depressions can be more severe than endogenous states, perhaps separate scales of severity need to be devised for these two broad groups of disorder.

4 Studies in Washington D.C., U.S.A.

From 1959 to 1960 Max Hamilton worked at the Clinical Neuropharmacology Research Center in Washington where he managed to develop further an important trial of chlorpromazine against placebo crossed in an elegant factorial design against additional social and occupational rehabilitation or none of these treatments. The results, important though unexpected, showed both drugs and social therapy to be efficacious but without any significant interaction between them.

Max provided an interesting but perhaps overdrawn picture of research workers at St. Elizabeth's Hospital in Washington, who were depicted as ambiguously poised between biological research projects in the day and training for psychoanalysis at night.

He failed to arouse any interest in his depression scale. The only journal that would accept the paper that described it was one that had his own discipline at the tail end of its title, *The Journal of Neurology, Neurosurgery and Psychiatry*. It took more than a decade before the HAM-D scale was recognised as a major contribution to knowledge and clinical practice.

5 Member of Medical Research Council External Staff (1960-1963) and Election to Chair of Psychiatry in Leeds (1963)

After returning to Great Britain, Max Hamilton spent 3 years as an external member on The Medical Research Council's (MRC) staff. He tried to re-establish his scientific studies at the local mental hospital where his scale had been developed, but this proved difficult and he conducted his enquiries under considerable impediments from an out-patient department.

In 1963 the Chair of Psychiatry fell vacant with the premature death of Professor Ronald Hargreaves. Max Hamilton estimated his chances as slender. However, he had made a habit over a number of years of visiting the University Staff Club where he found the company intellectually stimulating. He was contemptuous of hierarchical precedence, titles and honours, and tended to be iconoclastic and provocative in argument. But he was clear-headed, incisive and articulate and his worth and stature were recognised. None of his competitors could match his scientific knowledge and experience. He had also acquired a sound knowledge of computing and computer programming during the 3 MRC years – he had bought his first computer in 1948.

Max Hamilton was elected into the Chair. The establishment of a new curriculum for the teaching of undergraduates in psychiatry and the development of postgraduate education encroached upon the time he had been previously able to devote to scientific work. His wide clinical experience had led him to adopt a highly pragmatic attitude towards the teaching of undergraduates. The areas in which medicine had made large forward strides occupied little of the doctors' time. Most of the time of doctors in general practice in particular was absorbed in caring for those with chronic residual disabilities or conditions for which little or nothing could be done. It was among these problems that psychiatry loomed large. In Max's curriculum the clinical student was expected to acquire skill and had to learn how to make the diagnosis of the commonest psychiatric disorders and above all learn how to manage them. It was his belief that teachers of both undergraduate and postgraduate students of psychiatry would do well to begin by conceding their limitations rather than pronouncing their triumphs. The formula to cure sometimes, to alleviate often, and to comfort always remains valid even in the psychopharmacological era. But alleviation and comfort required intelligent planning, teamwork, a variety of clinical skills and insights and a personalised approach to the problems of individuals.

For his postgraduate educational programme, Max Hamilton conceived his department as being a community service station that provided trained psychiatrists for the region. His consultants were given joint appointments with local mental hospitals and their staff's teaching opportunities at the centre. It was a highly effective symbiosis. The three postgraduate courses catered for 20 psychiatric trainees and an equal number of those preparing for clinical psychology and psychiatric social work. It became one of the largest graduate programmes in the country.

6 Attitudes to the Role of Mental Hospitals

The facilities placed at Max Hamilton's disposal in Leeds – as in most teaching hospitals that created chairs of psychiatry – were scanty. Most of the scientific work he had initiated in the course of his career had been carried out in large mental hospitals either by himself or in collaboration with members of the clinical staff. Consultants in the neighbouring psychiatric hospitals were given honorary appointments in the Leeds University Department. In the 1960s and 1970s we met frequently and often discussed the problems looming up for psychiatry as a result of the proposed phasing out of the large mental hospitals and the progressive demoralisation of staff and the decline in the quality of the therapeutic environment that were already in evidence by the mid-1960s.

Until then there had been six special research units financed by Regional Health Authorities established at large mental hospitals. Their activities were not confined to laboratories or even traditional research pursuits. They played a major role in the creation of open-door hospitals, the tearing down of the gates and high walls of the old institutions and the development of experiments with various forms of care in the community. The presence of a team of investigators had set people on their toes and helped to sustain high standards of clinical diagnosis, care and after-care. Yet by the mid-1970s only two of the original seven units established within mental hospitals survived. At the present time no units financed by Health Authorities to undertake research in psychiatry remain.

A high proportion of the large-scale clinical trials into antipsychotic and antidepressive medication had been undertaken within the large traditional mental hospitals. Much of the clinical research on classification and diagnosis in the 1960s and 1970s, the follow-up studies and the investigations into the effects of social environment and familial background on the morale, clinical progress and quality of life of long-stay psychotic patients had also been developed there.

What was to be the fate of psychiatry as a clinical and scientific discipline when it had been deprived of its large hospitals and the land on which they had been established sold to property developers and farmers? That some required demolition and most of the others reduction in size and renovation was not in doubt. But how was research into the most recalcitrant problems of psychiatry to be conducted in the 30- to 50-bed units in general hospitals, which university departments are fortunate if they can secure. The "revolving door" which characterises the life style of acute psychiatric admission units is neither conducive to high standards of care and rehabilitation nor favourable to scientific enquiry.

7 Later Contributions

Scientifically, Max Hamilton's contribution in these years was the help and encouragement he gave members of his staff and other colleagues to undertake scientific work. He continued to pour out stimulating ideas to his pupils at conferences and meetings. He made fresh observations. However, Max had always been in the practice of doing more work than he published. Much of his research had in the past been undertaken primarily for the satisfaction of his curiosity. Formal publication was reserved for novel and important data. In 1974 he published his lucid and succinct "Lectures on the Methodology of Clinical Research" and in the following decade edited new editions of three of the books published by Frank Fish, a psychopathologist for whom he had considerable respect.

He was an early member of the CINP and a regular participant in its meetings and many other international gatherings, contributing scientific papers and, in his own inimitably sharp and challenging but kindly manner, to discussion. He was a stimulating and popular lecturer and travelled to many countries as invited speaker or visiting professor. His presence at meetings would always raise the level of arousal and enliven the atmosphere.

Max Hamilton's most lasting contributions to science have been his innovations in clinical trials, the development of his rating scales and the pioneering use of factor analysis and other multivariate statistical methods that had preceded them.

One issue implicit in his scales remains very much alive at the present time. Although it is clear from the items incorporated in his scales for anxiety disorders and depressive states that he appreciated the overlap between these two groups of disorders, he was departing from the unitary concept of affective disorders and gained influential support form workers of earlier generations such as Mapother and Lewis and younger investigators who followed in this tradition. The classification embodied in DSM-III and DSM-III-R allocated distinct categorical status to the anxiety and affective disorders. The controversy continues at the present time and it concerns theoretical and practical issues of wider significance. A number of workers have in quite recent years adduced evidence favouring the view that anxiety and depressive states are different points on a single continuum of disorders of affect. There are others who have advanced findings in support of a unitary concept of all the neurotic disorders, holding that not only anxiety and depressive states but obsessive-compulsive, phobic, and hysterical or somatoform and dissociative disorders are merely varying and transient manifestations of one and the same constitutional predisposition. This theory harks back to older positions of classical descriptive psychiatrists such as Kurt Schneider and Sjöbring and to the more recent concept of the "neurotic constitution" of Slater and of contemporary psychiatrists such as Tyrer and Andrews. On the other hand, DSM-III and its successors have jettisoned the concept of neurosis, judging it to be a redundant vestige of obsolete psychoanalytic doctrines. These and other basic problems of psychiatry will occupy psychiatrists in collaboration with other disciplines for many years to come. The various alternative theories will need to be submitted to stringent tests. Fresh clinical and follow-up studies will be required and the quantitative scales developed by Max Hamilton are bound to be used in evaluation along with others. But developments have reached a stage at which the tools of neurobiological science including those of molecular genetics will play a part of central importance.

A certain light is shed on part of the secret of Max Hamilton's success in his work with patients, whether in the clinic or in the course of enquiry, by some comments he made a few years before his death:

I found I became successful clinically because early on I cottoned on to the fact that it is not enough to see the patient; the relatives need treatment, comfort, reassurance, support, help and I spend almost as much time with relatives as with my patient – the result is that my patients take their drugs and come for follow-up. If they don't turn up I send a postcard: 'Sorry you couldn't turn up I am going to be there tomorrow' - and I go round to the home the next day. I used to be afraid that I would have the door slammed in my face. Nothing of the sort – I was invited in and offered tea and cake. My capacity for follow-up depends on my capacity for tea and cake.

With the passing of Max Hamilton, British and world psychiatry has been deprived on one of its most eminent clinical practitioners and investigators. A man of unusual vigour, and dedication to his subject, he made contributions of far-reaching importance to psychiatric science despite the facts that his gifts were late to be recognised and the facilities afforded him were limited. Drawing upon exceptional endowments of inner strength and conviction Max Hamilton was able to prevail in the face of prejudice, rejection and defeat. But for every one such person with just as much to give ten others are submerged by discouragement. Their thoughts may have been, in the words of the poet Gray, of "— purest ray serene —" but they are interred silent in "— the dark unfathomed caves of ocean". Original gifts are rare and they need to be recognized, nurtured and treasured.

Max Hamilton will be remembered for his courage and fortitude as exemplified during all his life to the very end. In my last meeting with him a few weeks before his death, he faced what he knew was a limited span of life with stoicism and tranquillity. He will be remembered for the refreshing clarity of his mind, the unrelenting force and determination with which he fought for his objectives, and the causes in which he believed, his delightfully impish sense of humour and the lasting affection he inspired in colleagues, pupils and patients alike. I hope his widow Doreen, whom we are happy to have with us here today, and his children and family will continue to derive some consolation from the knowledge that the work done by Max Hamilton will live on after him.

Acknowledgement. I should like to acknowledge my debt to information provided by Max Hamilton's widow Doreen. I have drawn also upon an interview with Brian Barraclough recorded in the *Bulletin* of the *British Journal of Psychiatry* in 1983.

References

Hamilton M (1959) The assessment of anxiety states by rating. Br J Med Psychol 32:50-55
Hamilton M (1960) A rating scale for depression. J Neurol Neurosurg Psychiatry 23:56-62
Hamilton M (1967) Development of a rating scale for primary depressive illness. Br J Soc Clin Psychol 6:178-196

The Hamilton Depression Rating Scale in a WHO Collaborative Program*

M. Gastpar [1] and U. Gilsdorf [1]

1 Introduction

In 1984 Bech and coworkers published a list of scales to be used preferentially in WHO studies in biological psychiatry. Among these, the Hamilton Depression Rating Scale (HAM-D) was the standard instrument for measuring severity and treatment effects in depressed patients, and has been used in WHO collaborative studies on drug treatment in depressed patients for many years (World Health Organization 1986). Furthermore, it was felt that the increasing number of new scales or instruments was inhibiting international communication rather than improving it, although versions derived from the original instrument, such as the Melancholia Scale (MES) by Bech and Rafaelsen (see Rafaelsen et al. 1980) showed better results in reliability studies, e.g., concerning the severity of present condition. This has recently been confirmed by Maier and Philipp (1985). A prerequisite for the proper use of a scale in a project is the training of the raters participating in the study. The analysis of such effects show that training is effective and learning effects can be documented (Bech et al. 1986). Difficulties can arise when studies last several years and it becomes necessary to replace raters.

2 Material and Method

The present data refer to a collaborative project studying the intravenous application of antidepressant drugs in depressed patients. A total of 135 patients were to be included in the study. Two centers, Bombay and Copenhagen, had to

*Prepared on behalf of the investigators from the WHO designated collaborative centers at: University Hospital of Psychiatry, Basle, Switzerland (Prof. P. Kielholz); Department of Psychiatry, K.E.M. Hospital, Bombay, India (Prof. V.N. Bagadia); Psychochemistry Institute, Rigshospitalet, Copenhagen, Denmark (Prof. O.J. Rafaelsen†/ Dr. P. Bech); Department of Psychiatry, King George's Medical College, Lucknow, India (Prof. B.B. Sethi); All Union Research Centre of Mental Health, Academy of Medical Sciences, Moscow, USSR (Prof. M.E. Vartanian); Department of Neuropsychiatry, Nagasaki University School of Medicine, Nagasaki, Japan (Prof. Y. Nakane); Department of Psychiatry and Neurology, Hokkaido University School of Medicine, Sapporo, Japan (Prof. I. Yamashita); Department of Psychiatry, The Medical School, University of Zagreb, Yugoslavia (Prof. N. Bohacek†). This study was conducted under the aegis and with coordinative support of the World Health Organization
[1] Rheinische Landes- und Hochschulklinik Essen, Hufelandstraße 55, 4300 Essen 1, FRG

The Hamilton Scales
Editors: Per Bech and Alec Coppen
(Psychopharmacology Series 9)
© Springer-Verlag Berlin Heidelberg 1990

be excluded from this analysis because of the small number of subjects. Consequently, 122 patients from six centers were finally included (Table 1). Despite the series of inclusion and exclusion criteria, there were some differences in the patient samples from the six centers – Basle, Lucknow, Moscow, Nagasaki, Sapporo, and Zagreb. In Zagreb, for example, only female patients were included, whereas in Moscow and Sapporo the average age of the patients was substantially lower (39 years) than the average age of the whole study population (44 years). The treatment effects of the first ten days measured with the HAM-D total score were analyzed with a two-factorial repeated measures ANOVA and revealed slight center differences ($p < 0.05$) and marked changes over time ($p = 0.001$). The interaction between day and center ($p = 0.0001$) indicates that the course of treatment effects differed substantially between the centers. Checking the average values of the HAM-D scores over time (Fig. 1)

Table 1. Characteristics of the patient population

	Center						Total
	Basle	Lucknow	Moscow	Nagasaki	Sapporo	Zagreb	
Sex							
Male	5	19	3	7	8		42
Female	11	12	27	5	4	21	80
Age							
£40	4	12	17	5	9	2	49
41-60	11	19	13	6	3	16	68
≥61	1			1		3	5
Mean	48.44	42.61	39.30	45.25	39.42	51.43	44.02
S.d.	8.68	6.40	13.14	12.11	8.87	8.36	10.64
ICD							
2961	15	25	26	7	11	16	100
2963	1	6	4	5	1	5	22
Total	16	31	30	12	12	21	122

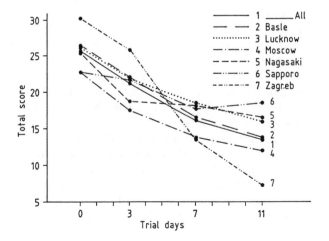

Fig. 1. Means of the HDRS total scores per center over time and means of the total patient population

shows that the significance of intercenter differences was mainly based on high initial values (Gastpar et al. 1985) and on a sharp drop in the scores during treatment at the Zagreb center. The main goal of the present analysis was to see if the symptom profiles at the different centers varied between center and/or over time. In principle, any differences might be based just on differences between patients or different rating styles; yet since group training sessions were held in each center before and also in the middle of the study, interrater differences should not be very significant.

3 Results

A visual inspection of the differences among the centers concerning the symptom profile given by the 17 HAM-D items is very instructive. Figure 2 gives the distribution of the severity levels of all 17 items (5 or 3 levels respectively) at four time points during the assessment, shown separately for each of the six centers. Comparing the initial scores, one can see definite intercenter differences at the beginning of the study. Basle, Moscow, and Nagasaki present relatively similar severity distributions at the beginning and over time for the first four items. In contrast, the other three centers present ratings extremely different from the others in at least one item, i.e., Lucknow in item two (feelings of guilt), Zagreb in item three (suicide) and Sapporo in item four (early insommia). At this point, we can only speculate whether the differences are influenced more by patients or rating styles, although both factors should have been excluded, at least to a considerable degree, by the joint trainings, initially conducted together for all centers and in the middle of the study within each center separately. Further examples for these differences are found, for example, in Lucknow in item seven (work and activities), where 100% of the patients were completely unable to do anything at day 0. This did not change very much until day 11. Similar symptom profiles were presented at Sapporo, whereas the Zagreb center shows 100% zero ratings in symptoms three, five and six at day 11, a fact that is completely different from all the other centers.

Considering these differences, it is still possible that the correlation between single items and the total score will be high, which means that these items would have a high reliability as long as well-trained raters are themselves reliable. An answer can be given by performing reliability tests using Cronbach's alpha coefficient. We then see (Table 2) that of the six reliable items found by Bech et al. (1981), three are included in the list of reliable items at day 0 and four at day 11. This means that – should they be omitted from the test – the overall reliability would be lower. Cronbach's alpha coefficient for all centers together on day 0 was only 0.48, but was 0.85 on day 11. Looking at the different centers separately and using the same analytical methodology, on day 0 four centers did not reach a coefficient of at least 0.50: Lucknow 0.13, Moscow 0.41, Sapporo 0.35, Zagreb 0.48. On day 11 all the Cronbach's alpha coefficients are at least over 0.60, ranging up to 0.89. The number of items increasing the reliability of the scale are between 8 and 13. Comparing the six

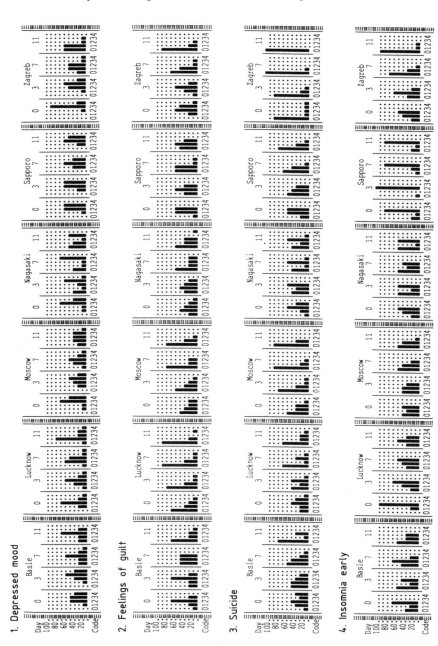

Fig. 2.a Distribution of the level of severity of items 1 to 4 of the HDRS, given for six centers over four points in time

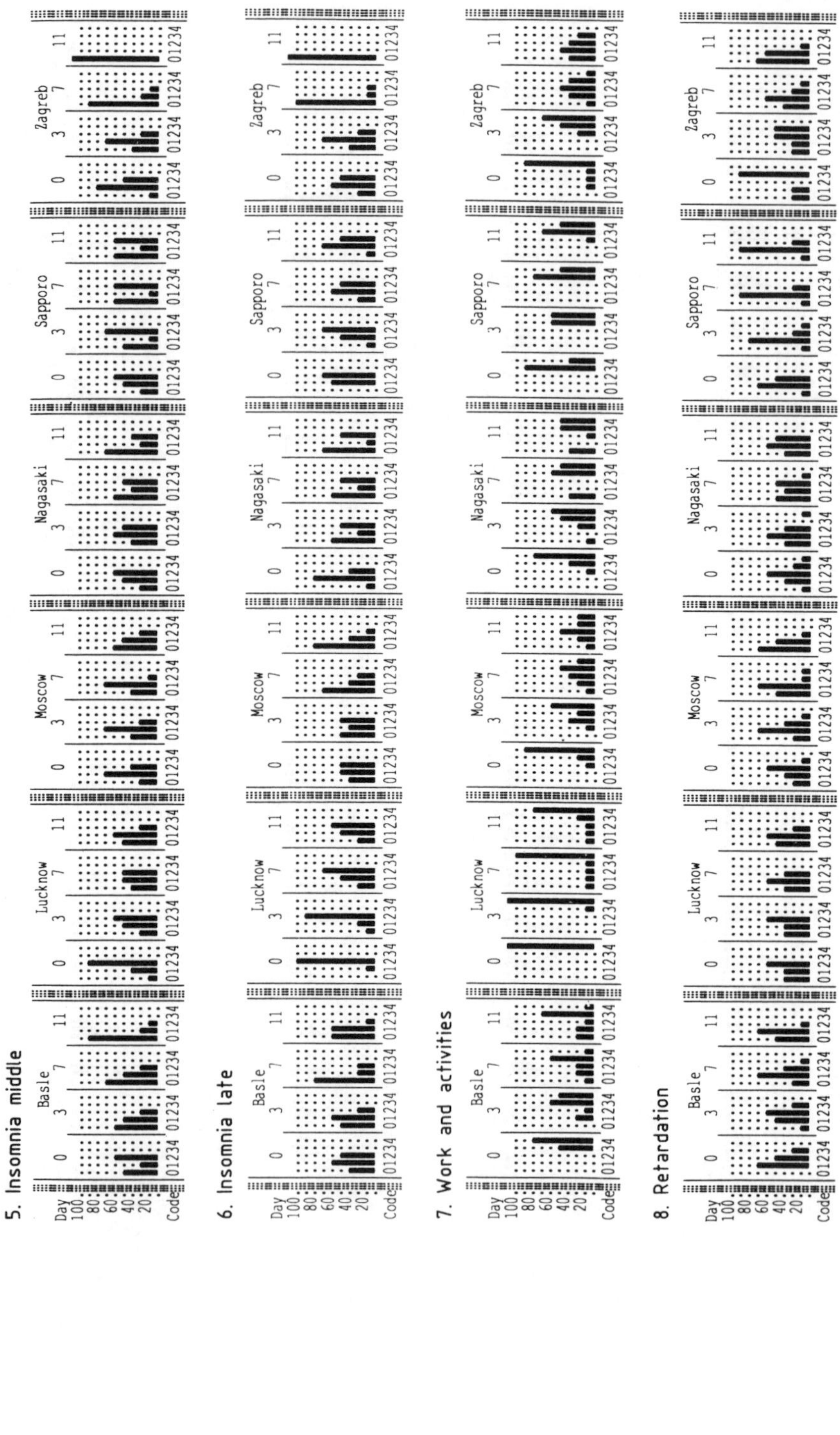

Fig. 2.b Distribution of the level of severity of items 5 to 8 of the HDRS, given for six centers over four points in time

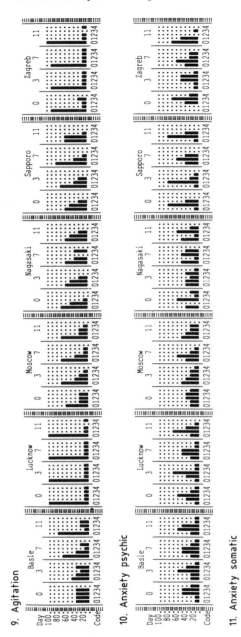

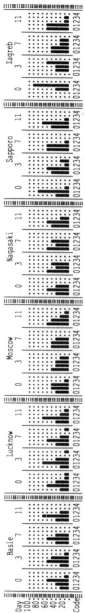

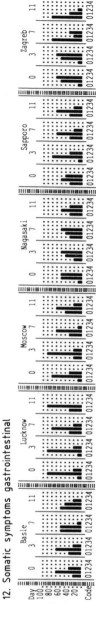

Fig. 2.c Distribution of the level of severity of items 9 to 12 of the HDRS, given for six centers over four points in time

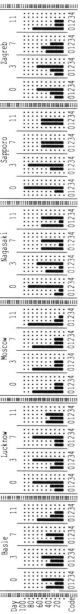

Fig. 2.d Distribution of the level of severity of items 13 to 16 of the HDRS, given for six centers over four points in time

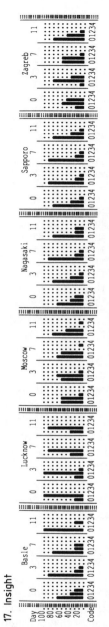

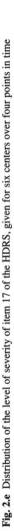

Fig. 2.e Distribution of the level of severity of item 17 of the HDRS, given for six centers over four points in time

Table 2. Correlation and reliability coefficients of all 17 HDRS items before and after a 10-day treatment

All Centres					
Day 00	Correl.	Reliab.	Day 11	Correl.	Reliab.
AnxPsychic	.39	.41 –	Work/Activ	.73	.83 –
AnxSomatic	.34	.42 –	Depr. Mood	.65	.83 –
Hypochond	.34	.41 –	AnxPsychic	.64	.83 –
SomGeneral	.32	.44 –	SomGeneral	.58	.84 –
SomGastro	.28	.45 –	GenitalSym	.55	.84 –
Insight	.25	.46 –	InsomLate	.53	.84 –
InsomMid	.22	.46 –	SomGastro	.53	.84 –
Guilt	.22	.45 –	Suicide	.50	.84 –
InsomLate	.13	.47 –	InsomMid	.46	.84 –
Depr. Mood	.10	.48 ==	AnxSomatic	.46	.84 –
Work/Activ	.09	.48 ==	InsomEarly	.44	.85 ==
Agitation	.07	.49 +++	Retardat	.40	.85 ==
GenitalSym	.05	.49 +++	Agitation	.40	.85 ==
InsomEarly	.04	.49 +++	Guilt	.39	.85 ==
Retardat	.03	.50 +++	Insight	.27	.85 ==
LossWeight	−.04	.51 +++	Hypochond	.23	.86 +++
Suicide	−.04	.53 +++	LossWeight	.11	.85 ==
	Alpha=	.48		Alpha=	.85

so-called Bech items (mood, guilt, psychomotor retardation, work/activity, psychic anxiety, somatic symptoms in general), the patients at the Basle center include in the list of positively reliable items five of six at day 0 and all six at day 11. Very similar are Moscow, Nagasaki, and Sapporo. At Zagreb, at both time points only four of the six items are included, whereas at Lucknow there are only two included at the beginning and five of the six items after 10 days of treatment. But all centers include a various number of additional items in the group of reliable items, so that there are considerable differences in item profiles contributing to reliability. Since the differences are strongly present on day 0 and are substantially reduced during treatment up to day 11, the treatment obviously equalized intercenter differences to a certain degree.

4 Discussion

In spite of the careful planning of this study, which included two training sessions for all the doctors involved, it is somewhat astonishing to see such large differences in the symptom profiles between six different centers that selected the patients according to the same criteria. The increase in the reliability coefficient from day 0 to day 11 during treatment suggests an argument along the lines that patients are initially quite different at the various centers and become more and more similar during the treatment. This means that the main difference between the centers is not caused by the rating style of the doctors. This can also be shown on a single item basis. For example, Lucknow and

Sapporo have an extremely high rate of patients completely unable to work or to participate in activities. At the same time, these two centers have the smallest improvement in the Hamilton total score, which corresponds well in clinical terms with the high severity of illness of these patients.

These results of the HAM-D total scores and the scores on the single items from the six different centers prove that the Hamilton Depression Rating Scale is partly reliable everywhere, although often insufficient. On the other hand, the scale can be used everywhere, because it is never completely unreliable. This situation could be one of the major reasons why the HAM-D is so widely used in the whole world, although the majority of the researchers complain about its lack of reliability. It can be assumed that highly reliable scales in a specific catchment area or culture would, in contrast, be very unreliable in a different cultural context. Thus we recommend that the HAM-D be used, at least in international collaborative studies, as an instrument which is applicable everywhere.

References

Bech P, Allerup P, Gram LF, Reisby N, Rosenberg R, Jacobsen O, Nagy A (1981) The Hamilton depression scale. Evaluation of objectivity using logistic models. Acta Psychiatr Scand 63:290–299

Bech P, Gastpar M, Mendlewicz J (1986) The role of training courses in multicenter trials: WHO experiences. In: Shagass C et al. (eds) Biological psychiatry. Elsevier, Amsterdam

Bech P, Gastpar M, Morozow PV (1984) Clinical assessment scales for biological psychiatry to be used in WHO studies. Progr Neuro-Psychopharmacology Biol Psychiatry 8: 190–196

Gastpar M, Gildorf U, Baumann P (1985) Comparison of oral and intravenous treatment of depressive states, a preliminary WHO collaborative study. In: Shagass C et al. (eds) Biological psychiatry. Elsevier, Amsterdam, pp 1503–1506

Maier W, Philipp M (1985) Improving the assessment of severity of depressive states: a reduction of the Hamilton depression scale. Pharmacopsychiatry 18:114–115

Rafaelsen OJ, Bech P, Bolwig TG, Kramp P, Gjerris A (1980) The Bech-Rafaelsen combined rating scale for mania and melancholia. In: Achte K, Aalberg V, Lonnqvist J (eds) Psychopathology of depression. Psychiatria Fennica Supplementum:327–331

World Health Organization (1986) Dose Effects of Antidepressant Medication in Different Populations. J Affective Discord [Suppl 2]: 1–6

The Impact of the Hamilton Rating Scale for Depression on the Development of a Center for Clinical Psychopharmacology Research

L. CONTI[1] and G.B. CASSANO[1]

All of us who had the opportunity of meeting Max Hamilton were agreeably surprised by his sense of moderation matched by his sense of humour. In spite of the widespread use made of the rating scales he created, and the fact that they are generally accepted as standard reference instruments, and in spite of the important role that these rating scales have had, not only on psychopharmacology but also in the fields of research and of clinical practice, he always retained a critical attitude. His philosophy and modesty are clearly shown by a sentence he used frequently: "I always check and firstly I check myself."

Because of our admiration and respect for Max Hamilton, we enthusiastically agreed to participate in this symposium; at the same time, we were frightened by the complexity of the topic we had been asked to speak on – the Hamilton rating scales in psychopharmacological research.

We considered various possibilities. First, we were tempted to present an accurate overview of the literature on the use of the Hamilton scales in psychopharmacology, but this did not seem particularly interesting.

Another possibility would have been to retrieve from our computer data bank the Hamilton scales for over 3000 patients who had taken part in psychopharmacological clinical trials. We could then have performed a series of sophisticated statistical analyses to demonstrate the usefulness of the scales and their value in assessing the therapeutic activity of antidepressant or antianxiety drugs, or their capacity to distinguish between the therapeutic spectra of activity of different drugs. But this seemed a celebration of our skill rather than a celebration of Max Hamilton.

In the end we felt that it would be much more suitable for this occasion, as well as much more meaningful, to outline the impact of the Hamilton Rating Scale for Depression (HAM-D) on the development of a center for clinical psychopharmacology research, such as the one in Pisa. I believe that our experience is very similar to that of many other centers and that the less young members of this audience will probably recognize themselves in our experiences.

The HAM-D has marked a step forward from clinical global assessment to the evaluation of psychopathological phenomena in their syndromic aspects. Since the purpose of this scale was that of "quantifying the results of an interview" (Hamilton 1960), its most appropriate application is to the field of

---

[1] Institute of Clinical Psychiatry, University of Pisa, Via Roma, 67, 56100 Pisa, Italy

The Hamilton Scales
Editors: Per Bech and Alec Coppen
(Psychopharmacology Series 9)
© Springer-Verlag Berlin Heidelberg 1990

research, particularly clinical psychopharmacology. But by using the HAM-D in these fields, we have also learned to transfer to clinical and therapeutic practice the analytical exploration of psychopathological features.

When a diagnosis of depression is given (and in that process we mentally refer to a syndromic pattern explored by the HAM-D), we try to establish the relative prevalence of the various aspects of depression in order to prescribe the most appropriate treatment, after which we evaluate the effects of the treatment not only as global improvement but also, and particularly, as improvement of the various aspects of the symptomatology.

The HAM-D was translated into Italian at the Psychiatric Institute, Pisa University in the early 1960s and it was used for the first time in Italy by us. Since then the HAM-D has accompanied our activity both in research and in clinical practice.

When, at the first national meeting of the Italian Society of Neuropsychopharmacology in Naples, we presented the results of our first psychopharmacological trial in which the HAM-D was used (Gallevi et al. 1967), it had a strong – either positive or negative – impact on the audience. Together with investigators who recognized the usefulness and the innovative features of this instrument, there were some others who emphasized its reductive nature and criticized its dissection and quantification of psychopathology.

Today the use of rating instruments is generally accepted and recognized as satisfactory both for research and for clinical practice.

For a long time now, the HAM-D has been the principal rating instrument used in clinical psychopharmacology and it is still one of the most important of them. It is still often used not only in clinical trials with antidepressant drugs but also, when the drug being investigated is an antianxiety or an antipsychotic drug, to verify its effect on the depressive aspects of the clinical picture or its potentiality for prodepressant activity.

The use of the HAM-D (and subsequently of the other rating scales) in clinical psychopharmacology, besides modifying the conceptual approach to the evaluation of the efficacy of psychotherapeutic drugs, has radically changed current methodological and operational approaches.

The use of standardized rating instruments and the quantification of psychopathology called for a statistical approach to fully and deeply analyse the collected data. This need induced us to acquire at least the basic knowledge required for statistical analyses and to set up contacts with statisticians in Italy and abroad. In this perspective we had fruitful contacts, outside Italy, with John Overall, Eugene Laska, Douglas McNair, and Phil Lavori. The considerable amount of information derived from the repeated assessment of patients during clinical trials and the increasing complexity of the statistical analyses performed convinced us that we should start using computers.

The creation in Pisa, in 1965, of a big university computer center, the CNUCE, gave us a great opportunity to utilize, right from the beginning, the enormous capabilities of sophisticated computers. At the Institute of Psychiatry, Pisa University, we created a computer center connected on-line with the CNUCE and much of its activity was devoted to psychopharmacology. The creation of the Data Bank for Psychopharmacology, the BDP, was the first important step. In 1977, with the help of Jerome Levine, at that time head of the Psychopharmacology Research Branch of the National Institute of Mental Health (NIMH) of the USA, the Biometric Laboratory Information Processing System (BLIPS) – an integrated system for data documentation in clinical psychopharmacology created at the Biometric Laboratory of the George Washington University as part of the ECDEU program of the NIMH – was installed in Pisa and integrated with the BDP (BLIPS/BDP).

At the same time, a Center for Clinical Psychopharmacology Data Documentation (CCPDD) was created within our institute, under the auspices of the University of Pisa and of the NIMH, with the aim of improving the methodology of clinical trials and the quality of data documentation on psychopharmacology (Cassano et al. 1985).

The availability of the psychopharmacology data bank, the BDP, allowed us to utilize the stored data from different clinical trials for methodological studies.

The HAM-D, the most important and widely used rating scale, was an important instrument in those studies. In 1971, for example, we presented in an International Symposium on Benzodiazepines held at the "Mario Negri" Institute of Milan, the results of an analysis on the HAM-D scores of 536 anxious or depressed patients – retrieved from the BDP – treated with antidepressant, antianxiety, antipsychotic (major tranquillizer) compounds, or placebo in different double-blind clinical trials performed according to comparable protocols (Cassano et al. 1973). The analyses showed that: (a) the spectrum of activity of benzodiazepines was characterized by "insomnia," "psychic and somatic anxiety," "agitation," "somatic gastrointestinal symptoms," and "work and activities" items, with no significant differences between the different benzodiazepine compounds; (b) that benzodiazepines could be differentiated from major tranquillizers because of their more valuable effect on the relief of anxiety and their better tolerance, and from antidepressants because of their greater effect on motor retardation and depressive symptoms; and that (c) benzodiazepines seemed to exert their therapeutic effect constantly on all neurotic and depressive subjects independently of their age.

Two years later we made an attempt to characterize the symptom pattern of elderly depressed patients on the basis of a quantitative cross-sectional examination of mental status, excluding etiological, prognostic, social, or dynamic considerations (Sarteschi et al. 1973).

A factor analysis of the HAM-D isolated three factors, the first corresponding to endogenous depression, the second indicative of anxiety, and the third expressing somatization (Table 1). The discriminant analysis performed on the factor scores was able to distinguish endogenous from neurotic patients mainly on the basis of the first factor of endogenous depression, and patients aged below 60 from those over 60 on the basis of overall severity, and prominence of somatization.

In 1979, with the aim of evaluating the role of benzodiazepines in the treatment of depression, we analyzed the HAM-D scores of 1057 depressed patients. Among the results, presented to the International Symposium on

Table 1. Rotated factor matrix. Items having a >.30 loading are reported (Sarteschi et al. 1973)

HAM-D items	First Factor	Second Factor	Third Factor
Depressed mood	.73		
Suicide	.62		
Work and interests	.62		
Retardation	.52		
Guilt	.49		
Psychic anxiety	.48	.37	
Depersonalization/derealization	.43		
Paranoid symptoms	.40		
Agitation	.36	.34	
Insomnia middle		.81	
Insomnia early		.77	
Insomnia late		.72	
Somatic symptoms, gastrointestinal		.37	.43
Somatic anxiety		.36	.50
Hypochondriasis			.59
Somatic symptoms, general			.30
Total score	.64	.44	.35

Table 2. Items included in two factors isolated by the factor analysis of HAM-D scores from 1057 depressed patients (Cassano and Conti 1981)

First Factor	Factor Loading	Second Factor	Factor Loading
Insomnia early	.56	Depressed mood	.59
Insomnia middle	.55	Work and activities	.55
Insomnia late	.53	Suicide	.49
Psychic anxiety	.39	Retardation	.49
Agitation	.39	Feelings of guilt	.45
Somatic anxiety	.38		
Somatic symptoms, gastrointestinal	.37		
Somatic symptoms, general	.36		

"Benzodiazepines: A Critical Overview" held in Brussels (Cassano and Conti 1981), a factor analysis allowed us to isolate two factors, the first of which included anxiety and insomnia and the second the core symptoms of depression (Table 2). In the clinical feature of depression, the load of anxiety appeared to be very high; the score for the anxiety factor was, in fact, greater or equal to that for the depression factor in 61.4% of the endogenous depressed patients and in 76.3% of the neurotic ones (Fig. 1).

More recently (Dell'Osso et al. 1988), utilizing the data from a large multi-center multinational prospectively randomized clinical trial in which the efficacy and safety of fluvoxamine was compared under double-blind conditions to imipramine and placebo (Amin et al. 1984; Cassano et al. 1986), it was demonstrated that clinical predictors of therapeutic response comprised the HAM-D items "diurnal variation" for both active treatments, "psychic anxiety" for fluvoxamine, and "loss of weight" and "loss of insight" for imipramine,

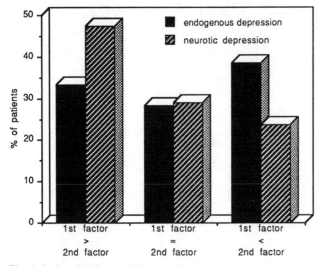

Fig. 1. Patient distribution (%) according to the higher loading of two factors representing anxiety (first) and depression (second), isolated by factor analysis of 1057 depressed patients' HAM-D scores (see Table 1). (Cassano and Conti 1981)

whereas nonresponse was predicted by "depersonalization/derealization" and "genital symptoms" for both treatments, by "retardation" and "somatic anxiety" for fluvoxamine, and by "gastrointestinal somatic symptoms" and "hypochondriasis" for imipramine.

To obtain a precise definition of any differences in patterns of therapeutic response to a selective serotoninergic antidepressant, fluvoxamine, compared with the most typical antidepressant, imipramine, we selected all the improved patients, adopting as a measure of their improvement a reduction in the HAM-D total score at the endpoint equal to or greater than 40% of the baseline total score (Conti 1989). The difference between the baseline and endpoint HAM-D scores of these patients has been factorialized with the exclusion of the insomnia items, since the administration of an hypnotic at night (mostly cloral hydrate) for insomnia was allowed.

From the three factors extracted (Table 3), it appears that the therapeutic activity of fluvoxamine is primarily exerted on the core symptoms of depression ("depressed mood," "work and activities," "retardation," "genital symptoms," and "suicide"). Secondarily, the improvement involves thought disturbances ("obsessive-compulsive and paranoid symptoms," "depersonalization/derealization," and "feelings of guilt"), "psychic anxiety," and – with a negative sign probably due to the gastric side effects of the compound – "gastrointestinal somatic symptoms". At a third level there is the activity on the somatization symptoms ("agitation," "somatic anxiety," and "hypochondriasis"), with a negative effect on the "diurnal variation" item.

The therapeutic activity of imipramine is primarily exerted on "psychic anxiety," "agitation," and thought disturbances ("obsessive-compulsive and

Table 3. Factor analysis on the differences of HAM-D scores between baseline and endpoint scores of depressed patients improved after treatment with fluvoxamine or impramine (Conti 1989)

Fluvoxamine		Imipramine	
Factor I			
Variance contribution: 42.1%		Variance contribution: 44%	
Depressed mood	.78	Psychic anxiety	.64
Work and activities	.67	Agitation	.63
Retardation	.55	Obsessive-compulsive symptoms	.61
Genital symptoms	.51	Paranoid symptoms	.52
Suicide	.46	Guilt feelings	.47
		Depersonalization/derealization	.46
Factor II			
Variance contribution: 33.6%		Variance contribution: 41.3%	
Obsessive-compulsive symptoms	.58	Depressed mood	.60
Paranoid symptoms	.57	Gastrointestinal somatic symptoms	.56
Depersonalization/derealization	.56	Suicide	.48
Psychic anxiety	.42	Work and activities	.44
Guilt feelings	.41	General somatic symptoms	.43
Gastrointestinal somatic symptoms	−.47	Genital symptoms	.41
Factor III			
Variance contribution: 24.3%		Variance contribution: 14.7%	
Agitation	.72	Hypochondriasis	.69
Somatic anxiety	.65	Somatic anxiety	.64
Hypochondriasis	.44		
Diurnal variation	−.46		

paranoid symptoms," "depersonalization/derealization," and "feelings of guilt"); the effect on the core symptoms of depression ("depressed mood," "suicide," "work and activities," and "genital symptoms") is at a second level and it is associated with the activity on "gastrointestinal and general somatic symptoms"; the activity on "hypochondriasis" and "somatic anxiety" appears at a third level.

Besides its use in psychopharmacology, the HAM-D has been largely utilized in Pisa for epidemiological studies on the prevalence of depression on alcoholism, on industrial workers, elderly people, and so on.

An important field of application of the HAM-D was an interesting experiment in cooperation with the general practitioner (GP). In 1975 a Center for Prevention and Treatment of Depression was organized at our institute and participating GPs in the area around Pisa were asked to call by telephone for assistance in the diagnosis and treatment of their depressed patients. To facilitate communication between the GP and the psychiatrist, the HAM-D, together with a Self-Assessment Depression Scale (SAD) by Cassano and Castrogiovanni, was utilized in order to describe the psychopathological characteristics of the patient and to define the severity of depression.

The choice of the HAM-D, was decided after a study carried out on 227 GPs in the area around Pisa (Cassano et al. 1974). These doctors were given a guided interview based on a questionnaire and were also requested to use the HAM-D in order to provide a profile corresponding to the depressive syndromes most commonly met in their practice.

The pattern of depressive symptomatology which emerged from that study was largely similar to the mean profile of 316 depressed patients assessed by psychiatrists, the differences being mostly related to the overestimation of insomnia and anxiety symptoms by GPs.

The activity of the Center for Prevention and Treatment of Depression lasted for approximately 4 years. It was very successful and contributed a great deal to the spread of the psychiatric knowledge among GPs and to the setting up of links with them.

Though rapid and largely incomplete, this overview on the use of the HAM-D at our center certainly outlines the great impact of this rating instrument not only on psychopharmacology but also on psychiatric practice. The emphasis I have placed on the HAM-D may appear to be excessive and obviously not all the advances made in psychopharmacology and psychiatry are due to this instrument. But it is certainly true that this simple rating scale has left an indelible mark on both theoretical and practical psychiatry. The HAM-D certainly has defects and limits but we can say with Hamilton himself (1960) that "Unfortunately, it cannot be said that perfection has been achieved, and indeed, there is considerable room for improvement."

The HAM-D has a limited coverage of symptoms, and some symptoms that are currently considered relevant to the concept of depression, like hypersomnia and fatigue, are not included in it. Even so, it has emerged as a "standard" measure of depression, probably thanks to its brevity and clarity, which largely compensate for its inevitable limits, and thanks to the universality of the language used. In fact the HAM-D should be considered a real international language through which we can communicate with psychiatrists all over the world.

I want to conclude with a sentence by Max Hamilton (1978) which provides a sample of his modesty and sense of humor:[1]

"Une échelle d'appréciation n'est rien de plus qu'une façon particulière d'enregistrer un jugement clinique. Le clinicien note son opinion sur la présence ou l'absence d'un symptôme, ou sur son intensité, mais qu'il la donne sous la forme de mots ou de chiffres, le jugement reste le même. Si le jugement est basé sur une information inadéquate, ou si le clinicien n'a pas une expérience suffisante, alors le jugement n'a pas de valeur, qu'il soit exprimé en mots ou en chiffres. Les analyses statistiques ultérieures n'impressionneront que ceux qui ne comprennent pas ou qui ne veulent pas comprendre ces choses."

---

[1] "A rating scale is nothing more than a special way of recording a clinical judgement. The clinician notes down his opinion on whether a symptom is present or absent, or how severe the symptom is, but whether he uses words or figures, the judgement remains the same. If the judgement is based on inadequate information or if the clinician is lacking in experience, the judgement is of no value whatsoever, regardless of whether it is expressed in words or figures. Subsequent statistical analyses will impress only those who do not understand such matters, or who do not want to understand them."

References

Amin MM, Ananth JV, Coleman BS, Dacourt G, Farkas T, Goldstein B, Lapierre YD, Paykel E, Wakelin JS (1984) Fluvoxamine: antidepressant effects confirmed in a placebo-controlled international study. Clin Neuropharmacol 7(s): 312–319

Cassano GB, Conti L (1981) Some considerations on the role of benzodiazepines in the treatment of depression. Br J Clin Pharmacol 11(s):23–29

Cassano GB, Castrogiovanni P, Conti L (1973) Drug responses in different anxiety states under benzodiazepine treatment. Some multivariate analyses for the evaluation of "Rating Scale for Depression" scores. In: Garattini S (ed) The benzodiazepines. Raven New York, pp 379–390

Cassano GB, Castrogiovani P, Conti L, Nardini AG, Viola L (1974) Recognition and treatment of depressive symptoms by non-psychiatrists. In: Kielholz P (ed) Depression in everyday practice. Huber, Berne, pp 174–183

Cassano GB, Conti L, Massimetti G, Mauri M, dell'Osso L (1985) CCPDD – un centro per la documentazione dei dati in psicofarmacologica clinica. Riv Psichiatr 20:1–17

Cassano GB, Conti L, Massimetti G, Mengali F, Wakelin JS, Levine J (1986) Use of a standardized documentation system (BLIPS/BDP) in the conduct of a multicenter international trial comparing fluvoxamine, imipramine and placebo. Psychopharmacol Bull 22:52–58

Conti L (1989) Predictors of response to fluvoxamine. ECNP Congress, May 24–26, Gothenburg

Dell'Osso L, Conti L, Cassano GB (1988) Imipramine, fluvoxamine and placebo: responders vs non-responders. AEP Meeting "Predictive factors of psychopharmacological response," Palma de Majorca

Gallevi M, Castrogiovanni P, Cassano GB (1967) Efficacia del Ro 4–5360 (Mogadon) nel trattamento degli stati ansiosi. Doppia prova cieca. Atti 1ª Riunione Nazionale della Società Italiana di Neuropsicofarmacologia, Napoli

Hamilton M (1960) A rating scale for depression. J Neurol Neurosurg Psychiatry 23:56–62

Hamilton M (1978) Les échelles d'appréciation dans la dépression: état actuel. In: Pichot P, Pull C (eds) La symptomatologie dépressive. Spires, Paris, pp 9–11

Sarteschi P, Cassano GB, Castrogiovanni P, Conti L (1973) The use of rating scales for computer analysis of the affective symptoms in old age. Compr Psychiatry 14:371–379

The Different Versions of the Hamilton Depression Rating Scale

F.G. Zitman,[1] M.F.G. Mennen,[1] E. Griez,[2] and C. Hooijer[3]

1 Introduction

The Hamilton Rating Scale for Depression (HAM-D) was published in 1960. Although many other depression rating scales have since become available, the first scale for the rating of depression severity has remained the most popular. Hamilton elucidated the meaning of the items and the way in which they have to be scored in a number of papers (e.g., Hamilton 1967, 1980). Of these, his paper from 1967 was the most influential. Hamilton himself never published a new version of his scale, i.e., a version in which the items are formulated in another way. Others, however, have done so. The first new version we know about was published in 1976 in the ECDEU Assessment Manual for Psychopharmacology (hereafter abbreviated as ECDEU, Guy 1976). This version differs from the 1960 version in many respects and several aspects are not in accordance with the explanations given by Hamilton in 1967. Nevertheless, in the ECDEU it is stated: "The present version is, we believe, the author's version." In 1985 Miller et al. published a Modified Hamilton Rating Scale for depression. Another version was published in 1986 by Bech et al. in their minicompendium for rating scales. Griffiths et al. (1987) and Williams (1988) published a complete text of the HAM-D as a structured interview. In our search using Medline (including 1200 titles), we did not find other published versions of the HAM-D.

In a process of standardization of rating scales used in psychiatric research in The Netherlands, it became clear to us that, at least in our country, a large number of versions of the HAM-D (and other depression rating scales) are being used which have never been published (Zitman et al. 1989). It also became clear that in many cases the version to which the authors refer is not the version they actually use. We decided to investigate whether this is a national (Dutch) or an international problem. To do so we asked the authors of papers published in psychiatric journals with a high impact factor to send us a copy of the HAM-D version they actually used in their recently published research.

[1] Department of Psychiatry, Katholieke Universiteit, P.O. Box 9101, 6500 HB Nijmegen, The Netherlands
[2] Department of Psychiatry, Rijks Universiteit Limburg, Maastricht, The Netherlands
[3] Department of Psychiatry, Vrije Universiteit, Amsterdam, The Netherlands

The Hamilton Scales
Editors: Per Bech and Alec Coppen
(Psychopharmacology Series 9)
© Springer-Verlag Berlin Heidelberg 1990

2 Methods

Issues of the *American Journal of Psychiatry,* the *Archives of General Psychiatry,* the *British Journal of Psychiatry,* the *Journal of Affective Disorders,* and the *Journal of Clinical Psychopharmacology* published between January 1987 and May 1988, were screened for research papers using the HAM-D. Of the papers fulfilling that criterion, we first looked for references to publications of the HAM-D in the list of references of the paper and in the paper itself, especially under the heading "Methods." We noted whether such a reference was given and which reference was given. We divided the articles into referring and nonreferring papers. Secondly, in a letter sent to the mailing address mentioned in the article, we asked for a copy of the depression scale actually used. After 1 month nonresponders received a reminder.

The actually used versions were used in two ways. First, we compared that version with the version to which the authors referred (if they referred to a version at all). Second, we looked for a published version which was most similar to the version actually used and compared them with each other.

3 Results

3.1 Reference to a Published HAM-D Version

The HAM-D was used in 93 studies in the journals during the period mentioned above. In 67 papers (72%) the authors referred to a published version of the Hamilton depression scale or to the paper published by Hamilton in 1967 in which he elucidates the way in which the items have to be scored. In 26 papers (28%) no reference to a published scale or to the 1967 publication by Hamilton could be found.

3.2 General Response Rate

A total of 51 authors (54%) sent us a copy of the scale they actually used. We will call them the responders. Among the papers of the responders there were 37 referring and 14 nonreferring papers. Among the papers of the 42 nonresponders there were 28 referring and 14 nonreferring papers. This difference is not statistically significant (chi-square 0.3787, $df=1$). In two papers a non-English HAM-D was used. We did not include these papers in the analysis.

3.3 Referred Version Versus Actually Used Version

Table 1 shows the concordance between the versions of the HAM-D actually used and the versions referred to in the papers. Only the first 17 items were included in this analysis. In only one of the 37 papers does the version actually used resemble the version to which the authors referred. If we include actually used versions in which some of the recommendations made in the Hamilton 1967 paper are adopted in the text of the scale, we find that the authors referred

Table 1. Referred and actually used scales

	Version Actually Used			
	Hamilton '60	ECDEU	Other	
Referred version				Total
Hamilton (1960)	1	13	6	20
Hamilton (1967)	2	11	4	17
ECDEU (Guy 1976)	0	0	0	0
No reference	2	9	3	14
Total	5	33	13	51

to the correct version in 5 of the 37 papers. In 11 papers the authors referred to the 1967 publication by Hamilton, but in fact used a scale resembling the ECDEU version. Because the ECDEU refers to Hamilton 1967, it is possible that the authors believed that the ECDEU version is, as is suggested in the ECDEU itself, Hamilton's own version. If we include these 11 papers, the number of papers in which the actually used version resembles the version to which the authors referred is 16(43%).

The depression scale published by Hamilton in 1960 and developed further in 1967 consists of 17 items for the measurement of severity of depression. He included 4 additional items for diagnostic purposes only. Eleven responders explicitly stated that they only used the first 17 items, while 19 responders sent us a 21-item version. The text of their scale suggests that they also included the last 4 items in the assessment of depression severity. One of these responders added another 6 items. It was not clear whether he used the sum scores of 21 or of 27 items. Fifteen responders sent a scale with 24 items. They included items concerning hopelessness, helplessness, and worthlessness, assessed depression severity, and added up the scores of the 24 items. One responder sent an 18-item version and five responders sent a 25-item version. In these versions the scores of all the items also were added up.

As is shown in Table 1, five studies used a version that resembled most closely the 1960 version, 33 studies used a version resembling the ECDEU, while 13 studies used another version. We will now discuss the differences with the original scales in more detail. We will confine ourselves to the first 17 items.

3.4 HAM-D 1960 Version

Five authors sent us a version of the HAM-D published by Hamilton in 1960. In only one of the corresponding publications did the authors refer to the publication of Hamilton from 1960. In two the authors referred to Hamilton's 1967 publication. In the other two no reference to any publication was made. They all followed not only the text, but also the layout more or less literally as it was published by Hamilton in Appendix II of his 1960 article. In one version, however, item 15, hypochondriasis, has been changed. Contrary to the original

Hamilton version, scores were attached to the description of the degrees of severity of hypochondriasis. The expression "Preoccupation with health" was replaced by "Much preoccupation with health" and was given a score of 2. "Querulous attitude" was replaced by "Strong conviction of disease" and was given a score of 3.

3.5 HAM-D ECDEU Version

Versions resembling mostly the ECDEU version were used in 33 research projects. Thirteen authors referred to Hamilton 1960 and 11 to Hamilton 1967. In the other 9 publications no reference could be found to a published version of the Hamilton scale. No two scales sent to us were completely the same. There were differences with respect to the scores per item, the number of scores per item, and with respect to the way in which the items were formulated.

In one version the score per item is not 0-2 or 0-4 but 1-3 or 1-5, making the minimal sum score on the 17-item scale 17. In other scales, the score range of only a few items is changed. In two versions the change concerns only item 3, suicide. In one version the maximum score is 3 instead of 4. In another the score range is 0-5: to score 4 is added, "any serious attempt rates 5." (In the ECDEU to score 4 is added, "any serious attempt rates 4.") In another version the score range of items 5 and 7 are changed. To item 5, insomnia middle (range in ECDEU version, 0-2), it is stated "any getting out of bed rates 3." To item 7, work and activities (range in ECDEU version, 0-4), it is stated "rate 5 if patient engages in no activities except ward chores, or if patient fails to perform ward chores unassisted." With respect to the score range of item 9, agitation, two groups of responders emerge. Eighteen responders use a score from 0 to 2, while 15 use a score from 0 to 4. This is probably caused by a contradiction in the ECDEU publication: item 9 is printed in the packet as a 3-point scale, but, as is mentioned in the instructions, it should be scored as a 5-point scale.

Now, let us analyse the description of the items and the scores. In one version the maximum score of item 11, anxiety somatic, is described as "sweating" instead of "incapacitating" as is done in the ECDEU. In the ECDEU examples of somatic anxiety are given. Nearly all versions use the same examples. Only two add a few examples to those given in the ECDEU: giddiness, blurred vision, and tinnitus. With respect to item 14, genital symptoms, nine responders had added "not ascertained" as an extra option allocating the score 0, 6, or 9. Especially scoring 0 can produce confusing results. In one scale the explanation about what is meant by item 14 is omitted completely, in another only the example "menstrual disturbances" is given and "loss of libido" (as in the ECDEU version) is omitted. These changes in item 14 suggest that in a number of research centers the investigators find it difficult to gather information concerning libido. In the ECDEU version there are two possibilities with respect to item 16, loss of weight. It states: "rate either A or B." In A weight is rated by history and in B weight is rated by actual measurements. In A as well as in B the score range is 0-3, in which 3 means, rather confusingly, "not assessed."

Only three rating scales are completely the same as the ECDEU version with respect to this item. The other responders use scales with a number of discrepancies. The instruction "rate either A or B" is omitted in 11 versions, but nevertheless a choice between A and B can be made. In three other scales not only the instruction is omitted, but also the possibility of choosing between A and B. In these three versions weight can only be assessed in one way indicated as "actual weight change" (in two versions) or "loss of weight." In one scale not assessed is scored as 0 which is just as confusing as a score of 3. Besides there are a number of smaller differences in the formulation of this item.

No major differences in the "ECDEU group" were found with respect to the formulation of ten items: 1, 2, 4, 6, 8, 10, 12, 13, 15, and 17. No version in this group was exactly the same as the version published in ECDEU.

3.6 Other Versions

There were 13 studies using a version which was characterized as "other." These versions are probably based on a combination of the remarks made by Hamilton in 1967 and of the ECDEU version. They did not resemble the versions published by Miller et al. (1985), Bech et al. (1986), Griffiths et al. (1987), or by Williams (1988). On behalf of the authors of nine papers, all working in the same institute, two versions were sent: the main difference between them being related to the comprehensiveness of the instructions added to each item. Because these scales were used in so many papers and as an illustration of the discrepancies, we will discuss these versions in some detail. The other actually used versions will be discussed only briefly. In the Hamilton 1967 publication no specifics are given with respect to the time it takes a patient to fall asleep, item 4. In the ECDEU version occasional difficulty falling asleep lasting more than 1/2 rates 1 point. In the scales sent to us on behalf of the nine authors, however, initial insomnia rates 1 if it takes the patient less than 30 min to fall asleep and 2 if it takes more than 30 min on most nights. With respect to item 5, middle insomnia, in the ECDEU version "any getting out of bed (other than to void) rates 2." In the versions sent to us it is added: "(same for smoking or reading in bed on waking)." Furthermore, it is specified that item 5 has to do with "difficulty falling asleep 12 midnight–3 AM." In one of the two versions it is also stated that, if middle insomnia is absent: "rate 1 if hypnotics are being used." In the Hamilton 67 and in the ECDEU version insomnia late, item 6, is not operationalized in a number of hours the patient wakes earlier than usual. In the versions sent to us the number of hours is specified in this item: the score is 2 if the patient "wakes 1-3 hours before usual time and is unable to sleep again." In item 11, anxiety somatic, the instruction in one of the two versions sent to us on behalf of the nine authors is, among other things: "avoid asking about possible medication, side effects (i.e., dry mouth, constipation)." Contrary to the instructions by Hamilton 1967 and the ECDEU, with respect to item 12, somatic symptoms gastrointestinal, no information about the use of laxatives is required. A last remark concerns item 17, weight loss. In the ECDEU version weight loss is specified as "greater than 1 lb weight loss in week" (rates 2) and "greater than 2 lb weight loss in week" (rates 3). In the versions we are discussing now, item 17 must be rated 2 if the weight loss (since onset of illness or the last 2 weeks) is less than 5 lb and it must be rated 3 if the weight loss is greater than or equal to 5 lb.

A third version has many items in common with the two versions described above. However, the definition of delayed insomnia (item 6) is different. One has to rate 1 if the patient "wakes earlier than usual, but less than 60 min or infrequently over 60 min." One has to rate 2 if the patient "wakes over 60 min before the usual time and is unable to return to sleep. This must occur more than twice a week or the patient scores 1 on this item." Here, the rater is not instructed to avoid questioning about medication with respect to the score of item 11, anxiety somatic. To item 17 concerning weight loss, specific instructions are added concerning the way one should assess weight changes when the HAM-D is rated more than once in the same patient.

We received another three versions, quite different among themselves, one of them sent by two authors. These three versions, again, are very different from the published versions. We will not discuss these versions in detail. Let us confine ourselves to a rather curious remark made with respect to item 15, hypochondriasis. To the maximum score, extreme hypochondriasis, is added: uncommon in men.

We analyzed the relationship between actually used version and place where that version was used. No two research centers could be found where exactly the same version of the HAM-D was used.

4 Discussion

The main findings of our study are as follows. If we are very flexible, 43% of the responders who referred to a published version of the HAM-D referred to the correct publication. If we are very strict, the correct reference was made in only 3% (i.e., one paper). Only four actually used versions were exactly the same as one of the published versions (the Hamilton 1960 version). We found many differences in the actually used versions all of which may influence the scores. This is true for the group of versions related to the ECDEU version as well as for the group with less clear relationships. The extent to which these differences influence the scores is unknown, because studies comparing one or more of the many versions we received have, as far as we know, not been carried out. In fact, no two research centers sent us the same version. To make things even more complicated, some studies used sum scores not of 17 items, but of more, even up to 25 items. The authors do not always report this. These results throw serious doubts on the comparability of the HAM-D scores in the papers we studied.

Is this gloomy picture an artefact of our method? We do not believe so. First of all, the response rate of 56% is quite good for such an inquiry. There is no indication that the 44% nonresponders are doing better. In fact, the number of papers without reference to a published HAM-D version did not differ between responders and nonresponders. Second, we have tried not to be too particular in our analysis. We did not discuss a great number of differences that seemed irrelevant. Besides, as we have already mentioned, research studies comparing these versions with each other are lacking as far as we know.

References

Bech P, Kastrup M, Rafaelsen OJ (1986) Mini-compendium of rating scales for anxiety, depression, mania, schizophrenia with corresponding DSM-III syndromes. Acta Psychiatr Scand [Suppl 326] 73

Griffiths RA, Good WR, Watson NP, O'Do.. .ell HF, Fell PJ, Shakespeare JM (1987) Depression, dementia and disability in the elderly, Br J Psychiatry 150:482–493

Guy W (ed) (1976) ECDEU assessment manual for psychopharmacology. National Institute of Mental Health, Rockville

Hamilton M (1960) A rating scale for depression. J Neurol Neurosurg Psychiatry 23:56–62

Hamilton M (1967) Development of a rating scale for primary depressive illness. Br J Soc Clin Psychol 6:278–296

Hamilton M (1980) Rating depressive patients. J Clin Psychiatry 41:21–24

Miller IV, Bishop S, Norman WH, Maddever H (1985) The modified Hamilton rating scale for depression: reliability and validity. Psychiatry Res 14:131–142

Williams JBW (1988) A structured interview guide for the Hamilton depression rating scale. Arch Gen Psychiatry 45:742–747

Zitman FG, Griez EJL, Hooijer C (1989) Standaardisering depressievragenlijsten. Tijdschr Psychiatr 89:114–123

French Experiences with the Hamilton Scales in Comparison with Other Scales for Depression and Anxiety

C.B. PULL[1]

1 Instead of an Introduction

I was quite young when I first met Professor Hamilton, at the occasion of a symposium on the symptomatology of depression, in Paris. Max Hamilton was to present a paper in French and Professor Pichot had asked me to help him in the French translation of his text (Hamilton 1981).

Hamilton arrived with a perfect French text of his paper. He nonetheless asked me to go through it with him, sentence by sentence, word by word, comma by comma and semicolon by semicolon, and insisted on reading it aloud several times, asking me to correct his French pronunciation in the smallest details. He was particularly interested in finding out whether the three or four "little jokes" he intended to tell would be understood by a French audience and was delighted when I smiled at the appropriate places.

When he had finished going through his paper, he patiently took his time to give me a personal lecture on how to make a presentation, emphasizing the need to speak very slowly, to look at one's audience, to know one's text by heart, not to develop more than two or three basic ideas, and, above all, to enliven the scientific speech with a few "little jokes."

When, later on, he delivered his presentation to the general audience, I could see that he did stick to the rules he had put forward to me, point by point. The remarkable thing about his presentation was that, although its written text was, by far, the shortest one in the whole symposium, it did contain and discuss the major points that needed to be discussed. All of the points made by Hamilton in Paris at that time, still apply today:

According to Max Hamilton, rating scales are used so extensively, especially in clinical drug trials, that most people will find it difficult to understand that they are not indispensable, even in drug trials. There are other ways to assess the state of a patient as well as the change under treatment. Among others, Hamilton mentioned duration of hospitalization and duration of leave for sickness.

According to Hamilton, the use of rating scales is nothing but a particular way for summarizing and coding clinical judgement. Clinical judgement is the

---

[1] Centre Hospitalier de Luxembourg, Service de Psychiatrie, 4 Rue Barblé, 1210 Luxembourg, Luxembourg

The Hamilton Scales
Editors: Per Bech and Alec Coppen
(Psychopharmacology Series 9)
© Springer-Verlag Berlin Heidelberg 1990

important thing, whether it is being provided in words or in numbers. When the judgement is based on inadequate information or when it is being made by someone who is not experienced enough, it will be worth nothing, be it in words or in numbers. Subsequent statistical analyses will impress only those who do not understand or who do not want to understand this matter.

According to Hamilton, available rating scales, including his own, are far from being perfect instruments. Concerning his depression rating scale, Hamilton mentioned that Per Bech had shown that the correlation between the severity of depression as measured by the scale and the severity as provided by global clinical judgement depended on only 6 out of the 17 items of the scale. Hamilton did not seem to be worried by these findings but did encourage rating scales specialists to further explore the psychometrics of existing scales and to develop new and better ones.

This paper is about the use of Hamilton's scales in France and, as such, no attempt will be made to discuss whether there are, at present, new instruments that are better than the ones Hamilton proposed more than 20 years ago.

Needless to say that attempts to beat Hamilton in this field have been numerous. Many new scales have been proposed for the assessment of depression and anxiety, even in France, although the French are not generally known to be frontrunners in the development of rating scales.

Widlöcher and his team (Jouvent et al. 1980) have developed a scale for the assessment of depressive retardation, De Bonis (1972) has developed a scale for measuring trait as well as state anxiety, and Widlöcher and myself (Pull and Widlöcher 1989) have recently proposed a scale for measuring the severity of inhibition in anxiety states.

None of those scales has, however, replaced either one of the two Hamilton scales. This does not mean, that the scales continue to be accepted without retraint by French clinicians and researchers. Both scales have in fact become the target of more and more criticism, but they continue to be included in most clinical drug trials, either alone or together with one or the other of the newer instruments which have been either developed in France or translated into French.

2 The Hamilton Scale for Depression (HAM-D)

The Hamilton Scale for Depression (HAM-D) (Hamilton 1967) has been translated into French by P. Pichot and his team, some 20 years ago. For reasons that are difficult to assess at this time, Pichot and his coworkers decided to translate a version which is not among the best known of the many versions which have been termed "official" Hamilton depression scales, either by Hamilton himself or by other rating scales specialists. It concerns an extension of the original 17-item scale to a 26-item scale, adding specific items for "diurnal variation of symptomatology" (item 18), "depersonalization/derealization" (item 19), "delusions" (item 20), "obsessive-compulsive symptoms" (item 21), "feelings of inadequacy" (item 22),"hopelessness" (item 23), and "devalorization" (item

24), and splitting 2 of the original items into respectively 2 independent items each: "diurnal variation" (morning and afternoon), and "weight loss" (reported weight loss and objectively measured weight loss).

It is this 26-item HAM-D which has been the standard HAM-D in France, during the past two decades, in clinical drug trials with antidepressants. Up to the present, the scale is systematically or almost systematically included in trials of this type.

Empirical studies on the scale itself have however remained scarce. To my knowledge, there are only two French studies which have been published on the scale itself, both in one of the oldest and most respected French journals, the *Annales Médico-Psychologiques*, a journal which appears in French with only a very short summary in English. Both publications are by J. Guelfi and other coworkers of the Pichot group and concern principal component analyses with varimax rotation of the 26-item version of the HAM-D.

In the first study (Guelfi et al. 1981a), computer simulations led to the conclusion that "2 statistically significant factors" could be identified in the scale, the first one a depression factor and the second an anxiety-somatization factor, and that "25 of the 26 items could be assigned to either one or the other of the 2 factors."

In the second study (Guelfi et al. 1981b), in which the authors attempted to replicate their earlier findings, use of more conventional statistical techniques identified 4 factors. The new factors did not "overlap with either those obtained in the first study or with factors that had been identified by other authors." Guelfi and coworkers conclude that "it thus appears that there is no such thing as a factorial structure of this scale."

The findings of studies concerning the HAM-D that have been published in the international literature have been reviewed several times in French journals during the past few years. In the latest review, which is to appear in the next issue of *Psychiatry and Psychobiology,* a journal which is published either in English or in French, but with extensive summaries in English, Cialdella and Chambon (1989) summarize the findings of a number of recent studies concerning the "unidimentionality" of the HAM-D. They conclude that no single replicable general factor has ever been found and that factor analyses and Rasch models are converging to the conclusion that use of the HAM-D global score is no longer justified." As such, and "en toute bonne logique," i.e., if we were to adopt a logical point of view, the global HAM-D score should no longer be used in clinical drug trials.

According to the same authors, "the Rasch model seems to support the validity of the Bech-Rafaelsen Melancholia Scale MES; Bech and Rafaelsen (1980) global score as a good assessment of severity of depression" and this instrument thus appears to be very "promising" for measuring severity of depression." Following those remarks, one would expect that the authors clearly propose that the HAM-D be discarded and replaced by the MES in clinical drug trials. Interestingly enough, no such statement is to be found among their conclusions.

3 The Hamilton Anxiety Rating Scale (HAM-A)

The other Hamilton scale, *the Hamilton Anxiety Rating Scale (HAM-A)* (Hamilton 1959), has also been translated into French by the Pichot group. In contrast with the HAM-D, which exists in several different versions, there is only one version of the anxiety rating scale. It consists of 14 groups of items, all of which have been found repeatedly to correlate positively with a general factor and to split quite nicely into a "somatic" and a "psychic" factor.

The scale has rapidly become and still remains the standard instrument for rating global severity of anxiety in French clinical drug trials, but, again, empirical work on the scale itself has remained very scarce in France. To my knowledge, only two such studies have been published up to the present.

Pichot and myself (Pichot et al. 1981) published the results of a principal components analysis on the scale. The paper appeared, in French, in *Psychiatria Fennica*. The principal components analysis before varimax rotation yielded three factors, with all 14 items positively and highly saturated in the first component. As such, we concluded that the scale was a satisfying instrument for measuring global severity of anxiety. Rotation of the two first principal components replicated Hamilton's own findings, in that the 14 items were clearly regrouped in either a somatic or a psychic anxiety factor.

The second study has appeared a few months ago in *Psychiatry and Psychobiology*. In this study, Widlöcher and myself (Pull and Widlöcher 1989) describe the development and validation of a rating scale for measuring the global severity of inhibition in anxiety states. Called WP2, the scale consists in 10 items describing different ways in which an anxious individual may be hindered, tied down, or restricted in his daily routine, and in which he or she has to make efforts which are out of proportion with the actual difficulties he or she has to face.

The purpose of this study was to evaluate the relationship between the degree of inhibition and the severity of anxiety, as well as their respective changes when treated with an anxiolytic agent. The HAM-A was chosen to assess severity of anxiety in comparison with degree of inhibition as measured by the WP2.

The distribution of global WP2 and Hamilton scale scores before treatment was unimodal and the two curves were superposable. In addition, evolution of average global WP2 scores was strongly correlated with reduction of global HAM-A scores. After month of treatment, average global score was reduced by 57% on the WP2 scale and by 51% on the HAM-A.

4 Instead of a Conclusion

There is no more to be said about French studies on either the HAM-D or the HAM-A and as such there is no need for a further summary or for concluding remarks. So let me come back to Max Hamilton himself. As mentioned in the Introduction, Hamilton just loved to put one of his "little jokes" into each of his presentations. One of the best known probably concerns a question he liked to ask his audience about what was needed to thoroughly evaluate a patient. He would look at his audience, wait a few seconds, and then come forward with "a bike," referring to the time when he went to see his patients at their home on his bicycle.

Well, I do hope that Professor Hamilton, from wherever he may now be looking at us, has put aside his bike and is enjoying the fact that his rating scales continue to be used and discussed.

References

Bech P, Rafaelsen OJ (1980) The use of rating scales examplified by a comparison of the Hamilton and the Bech-Rafaelson melancholia scale. Acta Psychiatr Scand [Suppl 285] 62: 128–31

Cialdella A, Chambon O (1989) The unidimentionality of rating scales. Psychiatr Psychobiol (in press)

De Bonis M (1972) Contribution à l'etude de l'anxiété par la méthode des questionnaires. Thesis, University René Descartes, Paris

Guelfi JD, Dreyfus JF, Rischel S, Blanchard C, Pichot P (1981a) Structure factorielle de l'echelle de dépression de Hamilton I. Ann Med Psychol (Paris) 139: 199–214

Guelfi JD, Dreyfus JF., Ruschel S, Blanchard C, Pichot P (1981b) Structure factorielle de l'echelle de dépression de Hamilton II. Ann Med Psychol (Paris) 139: 446–453

Hamilton M (1959) The assessment of anxiety states by rating. Br J Med Psychol 32:50–55

Hamilton M (1967) Development of a rating scale for primary depressive illness. Br J Soc Clin Psychol 6:278–296

Hamilton M (1981) Les echelles d'appréciation dans la dépression: état actuel. In: Pichot P, Pull CB (eds) La symptomatologie dépressive. Geigy, Paris

Jouvent R, Frechette D, Binoux F, Lancrenon S, Des Lauriers A (1980) Le ralentissement psychomoteur dans les états dépressifs: construction d'une echelle d'évaluation quantitative. Encephale 6: 41–58

Pichot P, Pull CB, Von Frenckell R, Pull MC (1981) Une analyse factorielle de l'échelle d'appréciation de l'anxiéte de Hamilton. Psychiatr Fenn Int Ed 9:183–189

Pull CB, Widlöcher D (1989) Anxiety-related inhibition. Psychiatr Psychobiol 4:1–11

Use of the Hamilton Depression Scale in General Practice

E.S. Paykel[1]

The Hamilton Depression Rating Scale (HAM-D) was originally derived on inpatients, and most of Max Hamilton's own studies were conducted on such patients. Depressed inpatients are relatively severely ill, and more likely to show psychotic or endogenous symptom patterns (Paykel et al. 1970). There are dangers in assuming that rating scales will behave with adequate reliability and validity in samples different to those in which they were developed. Very many outpatient studies have since used the scale and it does appear to retain its useful characteristics in these somewhat less severely ill samples.

In recent years the importance of depression treated in general practice has been recognised. In Britain the majority of patients are treated in general practice and only between one-sixth and one-tenth are referred to psychiatrists. A similar situation pertains in other countries with general practitioner health care systems. Even in the USA, where specialist care is highly developed and primary care less so, about one-half of the patients with milder disorders in the community receiving care do so from general medical rather than specialist mental health professionals (Schurman et al. 1985). Such patients tend to have mild depressions with different symptom patterns, and less evidence of endogenous symptoms even than outpatients (Sireling et al. 1985b). The majority of antidepressant prescribing is also in general practice, and controlled trials of antidepressants in this setting have become increasingly important (Paykel et al. 1988).

The Hamilton scale has, inevitably, started to be used in this setting. In setting up studies it is not uncommon to have reservations raised regarding the suitability of the item content. Thus, three of the items in the scale cover sleep, and others, such as retardation and agitation, disturbances mainly expected in severely ill, psychotic or endogenous depressives. In many of the individual items, there is only room for one point (at the most, two, in the 0–4 items) of abnormality at the level of illness to be expected in a general practice. However, little has been published regarding the value of the scale in this setting.

This paper will report relevant data obtained mainly from two studies of depression in general practice. The first was a survey study of depression, recognised and unrecognised, presenting to general practitioners in South London (Sireling et al. 1985a,b; Freeling et al. 1985). The second was a place-

---

[1] University of Cambridge, Addenbrooke's Hospital, Hills Road, Cambridge CB2 2QQ, UK

The Hamilton Scales
Editors: Per Bech and Alec Coppen
(Psychopharmacology Series 9)
© Springer-Verlag Berlin Heidelberg 1990

Table 1. Hamilton total scores in samples

	Inpatient (N=101)	Outpatient (N=118)	General practice[a] (N=167)	Three general practice subgroups[a]		
				Antidepressant treated (N=95)	Other treatments (N=48)	Missed RDC major (N=24)
Mean 17-item total	25.6	21.6	14.50	14.8	13.0	16.0
% ≥ 17	95	84	31	36	14	45

[a] From Sireling et al. (1985b)

bo-controlled trial of amitriptyline in general practice depression requiring antidepressant treatment, aimed at establishing which patients require and achieve therapeutic benefit from a tricyclic antidepressant (Paykel et al. 1988; Hollyman et al. 1988). For comparative purposes two other depressive samples will be used: (a) an inpatient sample, drawn from studies carried out between 1982 and 1988, comprising 101 depressives included in neuroendocrine and platelet-receptor binding studies carried out at St. George's Hospital Medical School, London and in Cambridge (Horton et al. 1986; Healy et al. in press); and (b) an outpatient sample comprising 118 subjects, derived from a larger sample in a controlled trial of phenelzine, amitriptyline and placebo, published some years ago (Rowan et al. 1982; Paykel et al. 1982). The studies were not designed primarily to investigate the utility of the scale and do not provide the full data set necessary for such an investigation, but do provide highly relevant data on selected aspects.

This paper will concentrate on three aspects: (a) the value of the total score from the scale as a marker of overall severity in different samples; (b) the make-up of the total score in different samples and whether the same items contribute; and (c) the ability of the scale to discriminate treatment effects in general practice.

1 Overall Levels

One of the most useful characteristics of the Hamilton scale is the extent to which the total score has been adopted virtually universally as an overall measure of severity, enabling easy communication to others of sample severity, and comparisons between samples.

Table 1 shows mean scores on the 17-item total (17-item totals will be used throughout this paper) for inpatient, outpatient and general practice depressive samples, the last derived from the survey study (Sireling et al. 1985b). There is a clear ranking, not in itself surprising, from inpatients to general practice patients, with all differences significant. There were three subsamples among the general practice depressives: depressives identified by GPs as being started on a new course of antidepressant; depressives identified as requiring treatment,

Table 2. Hamilton scale correlations of item to 17-item total

	Inpatient (N=101)	Outpatient (N=118)	General Practice (N=167)
Depressed mood	0.52	0.42	0.52
Guilt	0.31	0.38	0.41
Suicide	0.31	0.47	0.49
Insomnia, early	0.24	0.27	0.34
Insomnia, middle	0.21	0.34	0.35
Insomnia, late	0.38	0.30	0.34
Work and activities	0.59	0.58	0.59
Retardation	0.33	0.33	0.21
Agitation	0.37	0.20	0.25
Anxiety, psychic	0.53	0.33	0.50
Anxiety, somatic	0.41	0.47	0.42
Somatic, gastrointestinal	0.52	0.63	0.41[a]
Somatic, general	0.25	0.50	0.44
Genital symptoms	0.27	0.39	0.23
Hypochondriasis	0.33	0.43	0.16[a]
Loss of weight	0.40	0.49	0.42
Insight	0.45	0.23	-0.07[a,b]

[a] Significantly different to outpatient correlation at $P<0.05$
[b] Significantly different to inpatient correlation at $P<0.001$

but not an antidepressant; depressives fitting RDC criteria for major depression but missed by the GP and identified by the research team. For the third sample, the specific criteria selected a more severe group. Again, the discrimination by severity is informative, and patients selected by GPs for antidepressants are more severely ill than those given other treatment.

Table 1 also shows the percentage of the sample scoring 17 or more, a useful figure since it is a common inclusion criterion for controlled trials of new antidepressants. Only a minority of general practice depressives reach this level.

These findings are obvious and simple. Because of this, it is easy to lose sight of how important the Hamilton total score is as a standard tape measure for depressive severity, and how well this can serve when we step outside the familiar range. We all know the approximate meaning of a Hamilton score of 17, 13 or 26.

2 Item to Total Correlations

The potential problems with the Hamilton scale when used in a different range centre not so much around its utility as a measure of severity, as around its validity, and particularly, whether the make up of the total score might be greatly changed in milder patients, so that different items might contribute and the scores not really be comparable. To investigate this question correlations were examined of individual items with total scores calculated separately for inpa-

Table 3. Hamilton scale correlations of item to total of remaining 16 items

	Inpatient (N=101)	Outpatient (N=118)	General practice (N=167)
Depressed mood	0.41	0.34	0.37
Guilt	0.15*	0.21	0.41
Suicide	0.10*	0.32	0.33
Insomnia, early	0.10*	0.12*	0.17
Insomnia, middle	0.07*	0.21	0.20
Insomnia, late	0.26	0.14*	0.20
Work and activities	0.48	0.44	0.39
Retardation	0.16*	0.18	0.16
Agitation	0.20	0.09*	0.20
Anxiety, psychic	0.34	0.22	0.52
Anxiety, somatic	0.24	0.32	0.42
Somatic, gastrointestinal	0.42	0.52	0.41
Somatic, general	0.13*	0.42	0.44
Genital symptoms	0.13*	0.26	0.10*
Hypochondriasis	0.14*	0.27	0.04*
Loss of weight	0.28	0.37	0.27
Insight	0.32	0.15	-0.20

*Correlation fails to reach 5% significance

tients, day patients and outpatients. Findings are shown in Table 2. With the exception of insight in the general practice sample and agitation in the outpatient sample all the correlations were statistically significant.

Differences between item to total correlations of identical items in the general practice sample and each of the other two groups were tested for significance after z transformation. There were very few significant differences in correlations across samples: by and large the items contributing to the total scores ranked similarly in the different groups. Most notable among the differences was the lack of relationship of loss of insight to the total score in general practice: its contribution was highest among inpatients. In mildly ill patients it is likely to reflect aspects of self-understanding which are different from the absence of appreciation of illness, or occurrence of delusions, in the severely ill. Two other items showed significant differences only against the outpatient sample, although comparisons with inpatients showed similar trends. In the general practice sample, item to total correlations were lower for somatic gastrointestinal symptoms and for hypochondriasis. For the first, anorexia and constipation might have been expected to be less salient; the second finding was more unexpected. With these exceptions, the items tended to behave similarly in the two groups. The total score does appear to be valid on this very different population.

A better idea of the overall internal consistency of the scale can be obtained by using modified total scores, omitting the item in question. These item to modified total correlations are shown in Table 3. The scale does not comprise a single internally consistent total. Others have obtained similar findings using different analytic methods (Bech 1981). The least consistency was among inpatients, where eight of the 17 correlations failed to reach 5% significance. Among outpatients four did so. The scale was most internally consistent among general practice patients in whom only two correlations did not attain significance: hypochondriasis and genital symptoms. The negative correlation for loss of insight, which did not reach significance in the item to full total correlations, did so in this sample: patients with good insight tended to be more depressed, contrary to the direction in which the item is included in the total score.

The trend for greater internal consistency of the scale in general practice and outpatient than inpatient samples is consistent with other evidence that different areas of psychopathology, including self-reported mood, interview-assessed symptoms and social maladjustment, correlate better in the milder range (Paykel et al. 1973, 1978). It would appear that psychopathology and impairment are more global in this range.

3 Ability to Discriminate Drug Effects

The crucial test of a rating scale for psychopharmacology lies in its ability to detect drug effects. We used the Hamilton scale in a controlled trial of amitriptyline vs placebo in general practice depressives (Paykel et al. 1988; Hollyman et al. 1988). Two comparative measures were available: the self-report 90-item Hopkins Symptom Checklist (SCL 90; Lipman et al. 1979), and the Clinical Interview for Depression (CID; Paykel 1985) a 36-item interview scale, with 20 items used for repeat rating. Ratings were made after 2, 4 and 6 weeks' treatment. All scales were sensitive to change as judged by significance of pre-post change using the paired t-test.

Ability to discriminate drug from placebo was tested by comparing subtraction change scores in the two groups. The weakest scale in this context, surprisingly, was the self-report one. Its total score failed to show significant superiority of drug over placebo, and of its nine factor scores only one, for depression, showed significant drug-placebo differences, at the 5% level, at 2, 4 and 6 weeks.

In total scores both the Hamilton scale and the CID behaved well, showing drug significantly better than placebo at the 5% level at 2, 4 and 6 weeks. The CID has an anxiety total as well as one for depression and this failed to reach significance, at any point, confirming effects that were antidepressant rather than anxiolytic.

Often one wants to use individual scale items to obtain as much confirmatory evidence as possible as to target symptoms affected by a drug. Here the Hamilton scale has a well-known disadvantage: since the items are rated only on 3-point or at most 5-point scales, there is limited room for variation and precarious fit to parametric assumptions. The 7-point scales of the CID conveyed a considerable advantage here.

Table 4. Hamilton scale items showing significant drug-placebo differences in controlled trial of amitriptyline against placebo

	Week 2	Week 4	Week 6
Depressed mood	NS	<0.05	<0.01
Guilt	NS	<0.05	NS
Suicide	NS	NS	NS
Insomnia, early	<0.01	<0.05	<0.001
Insomnia, late	<0.05	<0.05	<0.05
Insomnia, middle	NS	NS	NS
Work and activities	NS	NS	NS
Retardation	NS	NS	NS
Agitation	NS	NS	NS
Anxiety, psychic	NS	NS	NS
Anxiety, somatic	NS	NS	NS
Somatic, gastrointestinal	NS	NS	NS
Somatic, general	NS	NS	<0.001
Genital symptoms	<0.05	NS	NS
Hypochondriasis	NS	NS	NS
Loss of weight	NS	NS	NS
Insight	NS	NS	NS

Table 5. Clinical interview for depression. Items showing significant drug-placebo differences in controlled trial of amitriptyline against placebo

	Week 2	Week 4	Week 6
Depressed feelings	<0.05	<0.05	<0.01
Guilt	<0.05	<0.01	<0.01
Pessimism	<0.05	<0.05	<0.05
Suicidal tendencies	NS	NS	NS
Work and interests	NS	NS	NS
Energy and fatigue	NS	<0.05	<0.01
Anxiety, psychic	<0.05	NS	<0.05
Panic attacks	NS	NS	NS
Phobic anxiety	NS	NS	NS
Avoidance, main phobia	NS	NS	NS
Anxiety, somatic	NS	NS	NS
Anorexia	NS	NS	NS
Increased appetite	NS	<0.01	NS
Irritability	<0.05	NS	NS
Initial insomnia	<0.001	<0.05	<0.01
Delayed insomnia	<0.05	<0.05	<0.01
Hostility	NS	NS	<0.05
Retardation	NS	NS	NS
Agitation	NS	NS	NS
Depressed appearance	NS	NS	<0.05

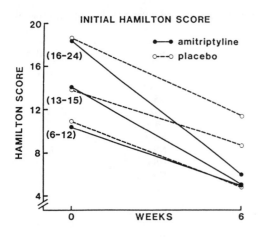

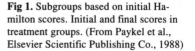

Fig 1. Subgroups based on initial Hamilton scores. Initial and final scores in treatment groups. (From Paykel et al., Elsevier Scientific Publishing Co., 1988)

Findings are shown in Tables 4 and 5. Only three individual items on the Hamilton scale reached significance as discriminators of drug vs placebo at 2 weeks, and four at 4 and 6 weeks: two at each point were insomnia ratings. On the CID seven items did so at 2 and 4 weeks, nine items at 6 weeks. Only two were insomnia ratings and most of the rest were core symptoms of depression, providing much better proof that the effect was a true antidepressant one.

A further demonstration that the Hamilton scale was useful was found when subgroups showing large and small drug-placebo differences were sought by seeking interactions in two-way drug by subtype analyses of covariance. Few interactions were found, and only when grouping was by initial severity, measured by RDC diagnosis major vs minor depression, or by initial Hamilton scale severity. As shown in Fig. 1, when three groups were formed by initial Hamilton scores of up to 12, 13–15, 16 or more, a clear differentiation was found, with drug-placebo differences absent in the mildest group, significant in the other two.

4 Conclusions

It should again be emphasised that the data reported here were not collected to validate the scale, but in the course of its use in different settings. Caution is necessary in taking scales further out into the world than intended by their progenitors, and, given the vagaries of scale and sample behaviour in any particular study, use of several scales rather than one is always prudent. However, the behaviour of the Hamilton scale in general practice depression is impressive. Its unique contribution is the knowledge of level that a total score conveys, in the context of widespread use in other studies. Within the general practice setting, this score is comparable in item contribution with its equivalent in other settings, and has greater internal consistency than among inpatients. The scale is sensitive to change in this milder range. Although the individual item ratings require supplementation when examining patterns of effects, the total score is able to discriminate drug effects, and the level at which they occur. Seen in this context, as in others, the Hamilton Depression Rating Scale has stood the test of time and constitutes a worthy monument to its creator.

References

Bech P (1981) Rating scales for affective disorders: their validity and consistency. Acta Psychiatr Scand [Suppl 295],

Freeling P, Rao BM, Paykel ES, Sireling LI, Burton RH (1985) Unrecognised depression in general practice. Br Med J 290:1880–1883

Healy D, Theodorou AE, Whitehouse AM, Lawrence KM, White W, Wilton-Cox H, Kerry SM, Horton RW, Paykel ES (in press) 3H-Imipramine binding to previously frozen platelets from depressed subjects before and after treatment. Br J Psychiatry

Hollyman JA, Freeling P, Paykel ES, Bhat A, Sedgwick P (1988) Double blind placebo controlled trial of amitriptyline among depressed patients in general practice. J R Coll Gen Pract 38: 393–397

Horton RW, Katona LCE, Theodorou AE, Hale AS, Davies SL, Tunnicliffe C, Yamaguchi Y, Paykel ES (1986) Platelet radioligand binding and neuroendocrine challenge tests in depression. CIBA Found Symp 123:83–104

Lipman RS, Covi L, Shapiro AK (1979) The Hopkins symptom checklist (HSCL): factors derived from the HSCL-90. J Affective Disord 1:9–24

Paykel ES (1985) The clinical interview for depression development, reliability and validity. J Affective Disord 9:85–96

Paykel ES, Klerman GL, Prusoff BA (1970) Treatment setting and clinical depression. Arch Gen Psychiatry 22:11–21

Paykel ES, Prusoff BA, Klerman GL, DiMascio A (1973) Self-report and clinician's assessments of depression. J Nerv Ment Dis 156:166–182

Paykel ES, Weissman MM, Prusoff BA (1978) Social maladjustment and severity of depression. Compr Psychiatry 19:121–128

Paykel ES, Rowan PR, Parker PR, Bhat AV (1982) Response to phenelzine and amitriptyline in subtypes of outpatient depression. Arch Gen Psychiatry 39:1041–1049

Paykel ES, Hollyman JA, Freeling P, Sedgwick P (1988) Predictors of therapeutic benefit from amitriptyline in mild depression: a general practice placebo-controlled trial. J Affective Disord 14:83–95

Rowan PR, Paykel ES, Parker RR (1982) Phenelzine and amitriptyline: effects of symptoms on neurotic depression. Br J Psychiatry 140:475–483

Schurman RA, Kramer PD, Mitchell JB (1985) The hidden mental health network. Arch Gen Psychiatry 42:89–94

Sireling LI, Paykel ES, Freeling P, Rao BM, Patel SP (1985a) Depression in general practice: case thresholds and diagnosis. Br J Psychiatry 147:113–119

Sireling LI, Freeling P, Rao BM, Patel SP (1985b) Depression in general practice: clinical features and comparison with outpatients. Br J Psychiatry 147:119–126

Structured Interview Guides for the Hamilton Rating Scales*

J.B.W. WILLIAMS[1]

1 Introduction

The Hamilton Depression Rating Scale (HAM-D) was developed during the late 1950s as a standardized scale for the measurement of the severity of depressive symptomatology (Hamilton 1960). The symptoms are defined by anchor point descriptions that increase in intensity; clinicians are to consider both the intensity and frequency of a symptom when assigning it a rating value. The scale was initially designed to yield a total score based on 17 of its 21 items, although many investigators have used all 21 items (Hedlund and Vieweg 1979).

Since its initial publication, the HAM-D has emerged as the most widely used scale for patient selection and follow-up in research studies of treatments for depression (Hedlund and Vieweg 1979; Carroll et al. 1973). Undoubtedly, the success of this scale is due to its comprehensive coverage of depressive symptoms and related psychopathology, as well as its strong psychometric properties (Hedlund and Vieweg 1979; Rehm and O'Hara 1985). In numerous studies, the total HAM-D score has proven reliable and to have a high degree of concurrent and differential validity (Carroll et al. 1973).

Since the HAM-D is commonly used to measure change over time, the individual items are often examined to study the differential effect of various treatments on specific symptoms or groups of symptoms of depression (Prusoff et al. 1976; Bech et al. 1984; Zimmerman et al. 1986). Therefore, reliability at the item level is important for research. Despite extensive study of the reliability and validity of the total HAM-D score, however, the psychometric characteristics of the individual items have not been well studied (Rehm and O'Hara 1985).

There are several studies reported in the literature in which the reliabilities of the individual items are examined. However, all but one of these studies reports reliability data resulting from joint interviews; that is, interviews in which one clinician interviews the patient and makes ratings on the instrument, and another clinician, *observing the same interview,* also makes ratings. In some studies the live interview was observed (Endicott et al. 1981); in others,

---

* A version of this paper appeared in the *Archives of General Psychiatry* 45:742-747, 1988; Copyright 1988, American Medical Association. This work was supported in part by Biomedical Support Research Grant #E759S, Research Foundation for Mental Hygiene, Inc.
[1] Department of Psychiatry, College of Physicians and Surgeons, Columbia University, 722 West 168th Street, New York, NY 10032, USA

The Hamilton Scales
Editors: Per Bech and Alec Coppen
(Psychopharmacology Series 9)
© Springer-Verlag Berlin Heidelberg 1990

the reliability ratings were made from a videotape of the original interview (Rehm and O'Hara 1985; Ziegler et al. 1978). However, because information variance is artificially eliminated with this joint observation procedure, it provides an inflated value for reliability if one is interested in generalizing to the real world in which different interviewers ask different questions to gather necessary information. Furthermore, with this joint reliability procedure, often the independence of the two clinicians' ratings is compromised when the rating decision of the interviewer inadvertently becomes known to the observing clinician because of its effect on the interviewer's inquiry (Spitzer and Williams 1985). For example, if in response to a question about suicidal ideation a patient describes thinking that sometimes he wishes he were dead, and the interviewer does not inquire further about any specific suicidal attempts, the observing clinician can assume that the interviewer will rate the severity of suicidal ideation as no more than mild.

Many researchers now regard the test-retest method as representing the "state of the art" of reliability assessment (Cicchetti and Prusoff 1983). In this procedure, two clinicians independently perform and rate interviews of the same subject, as close together in time as possible. The advantage of this procedure is that it more closely approximates the reliability of judgments made in actual practice, in which independent assessments are the rule. As expected, reliability obtained by this method is generally lower than that obtained by joint assessment because of the increase in information variance with the test-retest method (Spitzer and Williams 1985). Despite the fact that the test-retest method requires patients to undergo more interviews and may be more difficult to coordinate logistically, most researchers believe this expense is worth the increase in generalizability of the results.

The only published reliability study of the HAM-D in which the test-retest method was used and item reliabilities were reported was conducted by Cicchetti and Prusoff (1983). In this study a series of patients with major depression were interviewed by two clinicians at each of two points in time: at randomization into a controlled trial of a tricyclic antidepressant, and at the end of the clinical trial, in most cases 16 weeks after randomization. For most of the items only fair or poor agreement was obtained, although agreement was significantly better at the end point than at randomization, probably because of greater variability in the extent of depressive symptoms present.

This general lack of item reliability of the HAM-D may be due to one or both of two factors: varying interpretations of the meanings of the anchor point descriptions, and variability in the way in which the information is obtained to make the various rating distinctions. Many agree that certain items of the HAM-D are problematic and should be revised to increase their usefulness (Rehm and O'Hara 1985). Such a revision requires a major effort and is beyond the scope of this study. However, the current project grew out of an assumption that it should be possible to increase the reliability of the individual items by standardizing the way in which the rating information is obtained.

Since the availability of structured interview guides for rating various aspects of psychopathology, it has been amply demonstrated that the use of a structured interview guide generally increases the reliability of ratings (Endicott and Spitzer 1978). The specified questions in such a guide ensure that raters obtain the same information from all patients, thus reducing the information variance. This paper describes the result of an effort to improve the reliability of the HAM-D at the item level by developing and testing a new instrument called the Structured Interview Guide for the Hamilton Depression Rating Scale (SIGH-D) (Williams 1988a). It further describes other versions of the structured interview guide that have been developed for the Hamilton scales.

2 Development of the Interview Guide

The effort to develop a structured interview guide for the HAM-D began with observations of HAM-D interviews given routinely by a number of experienced clinicians. Based on this and the author's own extensive experience with the scale, interview questions were drafted that were appropriate for gathering the information necessary to make the various item distinctions in a relatively standard way.

For the purpose of this project, the version of the HAM-D that has come to be regarded in the United States as the more or less "standard" version was used (Guy 1976). Two very minor changes were made: under somatic symptoms gastrointestinal, the anchor point cues of "heavy feelings in abdomen" and "requests or requires laxatives or medication for bowels or medication for G.I. symptoms" were eliminated since they were cumbersome and were almost never used, and a note to code "O" if the individual was not depressed was added to the "insight" and "diurnal variation" items for individuals who had recovered from their depression or who were in treatment for another mental disorder and were not depressed. Finally, the order of the items was changed to better conform to the order in which the information is obtained in most clinical interviews.

Once the initial interview guide was developed, it was piloted on a number of patients from convenience samples. These included both psychiatric patients and patients with Parkinson's disease and depression, and included, in some cases, repeat ratings over time. In addition, the interview guide was distributed to a number of researchers who use the HAM-D as a routine instrument, urging them to try out the interview and asking for their comments. Finally, it was sent to Dr. Max Hamilton himself for his critical review. Revisions in the interview guide were subsequently made and repiloted on a small number of patients. The final instrument appears here as an Appendix.

3 The SIGH-D

The interview guide is prefaced by an information page for raters instructing them to begin the query for each item with the first recommended SIGH-D question (appearing in bold for each item). Often this question will elicit enough information about the severity and frequency of a symptom for the clinician to rate the item with confidence. Follow-up questions all provided, however, for use when further exploration or additional clarification of symptoms is necessary. The questions provided in the interview guide should be asked until enough information has been obtained to rate the item. In some cases, raters may also have to add their own follow-up questions to obtain necessary information.

Whenever possible, each area of inquiry begins with an open-ended question in order to encourage the patient to describe his or her experience in their own words. In this spirit, the interview begins with "I'd like to ask you some questions about the past week. How have you been feeling since last (day of week)?" The "depressed mood" item, then, begins with "What's your mood been like this past week?" and the insomnia items start with "How have you been sleeping over the last week?"

The interview guide was developed and tested for all 21 items of Hamilton's original scale, although Hamilton recommended that only the first 17 be used in calculating the total score (Hamilton 1960).

4 Method

In order to assess the effect of the use of the interview guide on the reliability of the individual items, a test-retest reliability study was conducted. Twenty-three patients were selected from the inpatient services of the New York State Psychiatric Institute. Patients were selected catch-as-catch-can based on the availability of raters and patients. Since several of the services at the Psychiatric Institute specialize in specific diagnostic areas, many patients were included in the study whose primary areas of psychopathology were eating disorders and personality disorders. Although not its originally intended use (Hamilton 1960), the use of the HAM-D in this study with patients whose primary complaint is not depression conforms to current use of the scale as a screening measure for severity of depression in the presence of other mental disorders (Halmi et al. 1986; Langer et al. 1986). Nine raters participated in this study: four psychiatrists, three senior psychiatric social workers (including the author, who participated in nine of the paired interviews), and two psychologists, both students in doctorate programs. All raters received 1.5h of didactic training that included practice rating and discussion of a demonstration videotaped interview, plus the supervised administration of the interview to at least one patient.

All test and retest interviews were conducted within 4 days of each other by clinicians blind to the complementary interview. Each set of interviews was followed within 3 days of the final interview by a discussion between the two raters to determine sources of disagreement. Of course, no individual ratings were changed on the basis of such discussion, even if it became clear that one rater had made a clerical error.

Table 1. Demographic and diagnostic information on study subjects

Sex		
Male	35%	(8)
Female	65%	(15)
Age		
Mean age in years	40	
DSM-III diagnoses:		
Alcohol hallucinosis and dependence	1	
Schizophrenia	3	
Schizoaffective	1	
Paranoid disorder	1	
Bipolar disorder, depressed	2	
Major depression	7	
Atypical depression	1	
Bulimia	6	
No axis I disorder	1	
(borderline personality disorder)		

5 Results

The average SIGH-D scores given by the "test" interviewers were 13.5 for the 17-item version, and 16.5 for the 21-item scale; the corresponding retest scores were 12.5 and 15.1. Table 1 provides the basic demographic and diagnostic data for the sample of patients evaluated.

The item reliabilities obtained in this study are presented in Table 2. Also presented for comparison are the reliabilities obtained in the Cicchetti and Prusoff study (1983) described above. As can be seen, nearly all of the SIGH-D item reliabilities are higher than those obtained in the Cicchetti and Prusoff study, in which an interview guide was not used. It is most appropriate to compare the SIGH-D results on inpatients with those that Cicchetti and Prusoff obtained at randomization into their drug trial, since that group would be more acutely ill than at the end of the trial. This comparison reveals that all but three (late insomnia, and psychomotor retardation and agitation) of the 21 SIGH-D items show better agreement. Compared with the Cicchetti and Prusoff results obtained at the end of the treatment period, only four (work and activities, late insomnia, psychomotor agitation, and diurnal variation) of the 21 SIGH-D items have a lower degree of reliability.

Of the 21 SIGH-D items tested, 12 showed good reliability (R=.6 or above). Of the remaining items, only two (work and activities, and hypochondriasis) had adequate variance in this sample to determine reliability. This lack of variance is undoubtedly due to the limitation of the subjects in this study to psychiatric inpatients. The total scores of both the 17-item and 21-item versions of the SIGH-D show excellent reliability, comparable with that found by Cicchetti and Prusoff.

Table 2. Test-retest item reliabilities of Hamilton Depression Rating Scale

HAM-D item	SIGH-D study (N=23)	Cicchetti and Prusoff (1983) At randomization (N=86)	At end (N=81)
Depressed mood	.80	.37	.72
Work and activities	.54	.33	.64
Genital symptoms	.70	.39	.59
Somatic symptoms GI	.59	.43	.51
Loss of weight	.58	.57	.06
Insomnia early	.80	.76	.57
Insomnia middle	.62	.57	.45
Insomnia late	.30	.42	.49
Somatic symptoms general	.61	.30	.42
Feelings of guilt	.63	.18	.37
Suicide	.64	.59	.64
Anxiety psychic	.78	.19	.40
Anxiety somatic	.66	.34	.45
Hypochondriasis	.55	.29	−.04
Insight	.00	−.02	−.03
Psychomotor retardation	.32	.39	.26
Psychomotor agitation	.11	.20	.32
Diurnal variation	.52	.50	.59
Depersonalization and derealization	.70	.15	.24
Paranoid symptoms	.74	.23	.32
Obsessional and compulsive symptoms	.87	.47	.25
17 Items	.81		
21 Items	.82		
22 Items[a]		.77	.89

[a] Total score calculated on 22 items because diurnal variation and diurnal variation (severe) were considered separate items

The HAM-D scale alone requires at least a 1/2 h to administer (Hamilton 1967). Raters in this study were asked to note the amount of time each SIGH-D interview took. The average amount of time was 28 min, indicating that the use of the SIGH-D does not increase the amount of time necessary to administer the scale over routine use.

6 Discussion

This study demonstrates that the use of a structured interview guide for the HAM-D results in generally increased reliability at the item level. This is similar to what was demonstrated by Endicott et al. (Endicott et al. 1981) in a comparison of agreement obtained by joint interviews on items from the Schedule for Affective Disorders and Schizophrenia — Change Version (SADS-C) that were similar to the HAM-D items, and agreement on items from the actual

HAM-D scale. That study also demonstrated better agreement using the structured interview guide, although it was not developed specifically for rating the HAM-D items.

All but two of the raters in the SIGH-D study had not had any experience with the HAM-D prior to this study. The increase in item reliability with the SIGH-D is all the more impressive given the minimal training the interviewers received, the fact that they were of disparate backgrounds, and that for the most part they had not worked together before. This suggests that the SIGH-D may be an efficient way to incorporate new raters quickly into a research program that uses the HAM-D, without sacrificing reliability. This study also demonstrates that the use of this interview guide does not increase the amount of time necessary to administer the scale over routine clinical use.

Ideally, this study would have compared the test-retest reliability of the HAM-D as usually administered (i.e., without an interview guide), with the test-retest reliability of the SIGH-D, on the same sample of subjects. However, such a study design would have involved administering the scale four times to each subject, a plan that is obviously not without its own logistic and scientific drawbacks. For this reason, the Cicchetti and Prusoff study was used as the comparison measure, with the recognition that since it involved a different sample of subjects, it is not the ideal control group.

Many critiques have been written of the HAM-D citing difficulties with the items ranging from lack of specificity of the item descriptions to poor discriminative validity of the individual items (Cicchetti and Prusoff 1983; Miller et al. 1985). And unfortunately, although they are improved, in general the item reliabilities even using the SIGH-D are still not what one would hope. Only half of them are in the excellent to good range, with the rest ranging from fair to poor. This study was not designed to improve on the HAM-D, but rather to improve the reliability of the original scale items.

7 Other Interview Guides for the Hamilton Scales

Bolstered by the increase in item reliability that apparently results from the use of an interview guide, the author developed a similar guide for the Hamilton Anxiety Rating Scale (HAM-A; Hamilton 1959). Because of the overlap in item content of the HAM-D and the HAM-A, and the usual need to assess both anxiety and depressive symptoms, the interview guides for the two scales have been combined into the SIGH-AD (Structured Interview Guide for the Hamilton Anxiety and Depression Rating Scales; Williams 1988b). Although the SIGH-AD has not yet been subjected to formal reliability testing, it is currently being used in several studies.

Researchers studying treatments for the recently recognized syndrome of seasonal affective disorder generally assess changes in the severity of depressive symptoms at weekly visits. Eight items (and corresponding interview questions) describing special features of the seasonal syndrome have been added to the SIGH-D, and the resulting SIGH-SAD (Structured Interview Guide for the

Hamilton Depression Rating Scale — Seasonal Affective Disorders Version; Williams et al. 1988a) is used as a standard assessment tool in many studies in this area. Plans are now under way to conduct a formal reliability test of the SIGH-SAD. In addition, because of the need in this field to examine hypomanic symptoms when patients are not depressed, the HIGH-SAD (Hypomania Interview Guide (including Hyperthymia) for Seasonal Affective Disorder; Williams et al. 1988b) has been developed.

Acknowledgements. The author would like to thank the raters in the reliability study, Mss. Miriam Gibbon, Mary Sano, Joan Carrillo, Jo Ellen Loth, and Drs. Robert Aranow, Michael First, Lawrence Jacobsberg, and Ronald Winchell, research assistant Raymond Henriques, statistical consultant Mark Davies, and critical reviewer Dr. Robert Spitzer.

References

Bech P, Allerup P, Reisby N, Gram LF (1984) Assessment of symptoms change from improvement curves on the Hamilton depression scale in trials with antidepressants. Psychopharmacology (Berlin) 84:276–281

Carroll BJ, Fielding JM, Blashki TG (1973) Depression rating scales: a critical review. Arch Gen Psychiatry 28:361–366

Cicchetti DV, Prusoff BA (1983) Reliability of depression and associated clinical symptoms. Arch Gen Psychiatry 40:987–990

Endicott J Spitzer RL (1978) A diagnostic interview: the schedule for affective disorders and schizophrenia. Arch Gen Psychiatry 35:837–844

Endicott J, Cohen J, Nee J et al. (1981) Hamilton depression rating scale: extracted from regular and change versions of the schedule for affective disorders and schizophrenia. Arch Gen Psychiatry 38:98–103

Guy W (ed) (1976) ECDEU assessment manual for psychopharmacology, no ADM 76–336. US Department of Health, Education, and Welfare, Rockville

Halmi KA, Eckert E, LaDu TJ, Cohen J (1986) Anorexia nervosa: treatment efficacy of cyproheptadine and amitriptyline. Arch Gen Psychiatry 43:177–181

Hamilton M (1959) The assessment of anxiety states by rating. Br J Med Psychol 32:50–55

Hamilton M (1960) A rating scale for depression. J Neurol Neurosurg Psychiatry 23:56–62

Hamilton M (1967) Development of a rating scale for primary depressive illness. Br J Soc Clin Psychol 6:278–296

Hedlund JL, Vieweg BW (1979) The Hamilton rating scale for depression: a comprehensive review. J Operat Psychiatry 10:149–165

Langer G, Koinig G, Hatzinger R, Schonbeck G, Resch F, Aschauer H, Keshavan MS, Sieghart W (1986) Response of thyrotropin to thyrotropin-releasing hormone as predictor of treatment outcome: prediction of recovery and relapse in treatment with antidepressants and neuroleptics. Arch Gen Psychiatry 43:861–868

Miller IW, Bishop S, Norman WH, Maddever H (1985) The modified Hamilton rating scale for depression: reliability and validity. Psychiatry Res 14:131–142

Prusoff BA, Weissman M, Tanner J et al. (1976) Symptom reduction in depressed outpatients treated with amitriptyline or maprotiline: repeated measurement analysis. Compr Psychiatry 17:749–754

Rehm LP, O'Hara MW (1985) Item characteristics of the Hamilton rating scale for depression. J Psychiatr Res 19:31–41

Spitzer RL, Williams JBW (1985) Classification in psychiatry. In: Kaplan H, Sadock B (eds) Comprehensive textbook of psychiatry, 4th edn. Williams and Wilkins, Baltimore, pp 591–613

Williams JBW (1988a) A structured interview guide for the Hamilton depression rating scale. Arch Gen Psychiatry 45:742–747

Williams JBW (1988b) Structured interview guide for the Hamilton anxiety and depression rating scales (SIGH-AD). New York State Psychiatric Institute, New York

Williams JBW, Link MJ, Rosenthal N, Terman M (1988a) Structured interview guide for the Hamilton depression rating scale – seasonal affective disorders version (SIGH-SAD). New York State Psychiatric Institute, New York

Williams JBW, Link MJ, Rosenthal NE, Terman M (1988b) Hypomania interview guide (including hyperthymia) for seasonal affective disorder (HIGH-SAD). New York State Psychiatric Institute, New York

Ziegler VE, Meyer DA, Rosen SH, Biggs JT (1978) Reliability of video taped Hamilton ratings. Biol Psychiatry 13:119–122

Zimmerman M, Coryell W, Pfhol B, Stangl D (1986) Validity of the Hamilton endogenous subscale: an independent replication. Psychiatry Res 18:209–215

Appendix. Structured Interview Guide for the Hamilton Depression Rating Scale (SIGH-D)*

Introduction

Interviewer

The first question for each item should be asked exactly as written. Often this question will elicit enough information about the severity and frequency of a symptom for you to rate the item with confidence. Follow-up questions are provided, however, for use when further exploration or additional clarification of symptoms is necessary. The specified questions should be asked until you have enough information to rate the item confidently. In some cases, you may also have to add your own follow-up questions to obtain necessary information.

Notes

Time period. Although the interview questions indicate that the ratings should be based on the patient's condition in the past week, some investigators using this instrument as a change measure may wish to base their ratings on the previous 2 to 3 days. If so, the questions may be preceded by "In the last couple of days...."

Loss of weight item. It is recommended that this item be rated positively whenever the patient has lost weight relative to their baseline weight (i.e., before their current episode of depression), provided that they have not begun to gain back lost weight. Once the patient has begun to gain weight, however, even if they are still below their baseline, they should no longer be rated positively on this item.

Referent of "usual" or "normal" condition. Several of the interview questions refer to the patient's usual or normal functioning. In some cases, such as when the patient has Dysthymia or Seasonal Affective Disorder, the referent should be to the last time they felt OK (i.e., not depressed or high) for at least a few weeks.

This interview guide is based on the Hamilton Depression Rating Scale (Hamilton 1960). The anchor point descriptions, with very minor modifications, have been taken from the ECDEU Assessment Manual (Guy 1976).

* This work was supported in part by Biomedical Research Support Grant #903-E759S from the Research Foundation for Mental Hygiene, Inc.

Interview[1]

Pt's name: _____ Pt's ID: _____ (1-7)

Interviewer: _____ Date: _____ (8-13)

Overview: I'd like to ask you some questions about the past week. How have you been feeling since last (day of week)? If outpatient: Have you been working? If not: Why not?

What's your mood been like this past week?

Have you been feeling down or depressed?

Sad? Hopeless?

In the last week, how often have you felt (Own equivalent)? Every day? All day?

Have you been crying at all?

Depressed mood (sadness, hopeless, helpless, worthless):

0 – Absent
1 – Indicated only on questioning
2 – Spontaneously reported verbally
3 – Communicated nonverbally, i.e., facial expression, posture, voice, tendency to weep
4 – Virtually only; this in spontaneous verbal and nonverbal communication   (15)

If scored 1–4 above, ask: How long have you been feeling this way?

How have you been spending your time this past week (when not at work)?

Have you felt interested in doing (those things), or do you feel you have to push yourself to do them?

Have you stopped doing anything you used to do? *If yes:* Why?

Is there anything you look forward to?

(At follow-up: Has your interest been back to normal?)

Work and Activities:

0 – No difficulty
1 – Thoughts and feelings of incapacity, fatigue, or weakness related to activities, work, or hobbies
2 – Loss of interest in activity, hobbies or work – by direct report of the patient or indirect in listlessness, indecision, and vacillation (feels he has to push self to work or activities)
3 – Decrease in actual time spent in activities or decrease in productivity. In hosp, pt. spends less than 3 h/day in activities (hospital job or hobbies) exclusive of ward chores
4 – Stopped working because of present illness. In hospital, no activities except ward chores, or fails to perform ward chores unassisted   (16)

---

[1] Prepared by Janet B.W. Williams, D.S.W. Biometrics Research Department, New York State Psychiatric Institute, 722 West 168th Street, New York, NY 10032, USA

How has your interest in sex been this week?

Has there been any change in your interest in sex (from when you were not depressed)?

Is it something you've thought much about? IF NO: Is that unusual for you?

Genital Symptoms (such as loss of libido, menstrual disturbances):

0 – Absent
1 – Mild
2 – Severe (17)

How has your appetite been this past week? (What about compared to your usual appetite?)

Have you had to force yourself to eat?

Have other people had to urge you to eat?

Somatic Symptoms Gastrointestinal:

0 – None
1 – Loss of appetite but eating without encouragement
2 – Difficulty eating without urging (18)

Have you lost any weight since this (Depression) began? IF YES: How much?

If not sure: Do you think your clothes are any looser on you?

At follow-up: Have you gained any of the weight back?

Loss Of Weight (Rate either A or B):

A. When rating by history:
0 – No weight loss
1 – Probable weight loss associated with present illness
2 – Definite (according to patient) weight loss
3 – Not assessed (19)

B. On weekly ratings by ward staff, when actual weight changes are measured:

0 – Less than 1 lb loss in week
1 – More than 1 lb loss in week
2 – More than 2 lbs loss in week
3 – Not assessed (20)

How have you been sleeping over the last week?

Have you had any trouble falling asleep at the beginning of the night?

(Right after you go to bed, how long has it been taking you to fall asleep?)

How many nights this week have you had trouble falling asleep?

Insomnia Early:

0 – No difficulty falling asleep
1 – Complains of occasional difficulty falling asleep – i.e., more than 1/2 h
2 – Complains of nightly difficulty falling asleep (21)

During the past week, have you been waking up in the middle of the night?

If yes: Do you get out of bed? What do you do? (Only go to the bathroom?)

When you get back in bed, are you able to fall right back asleep?

Have you felt your sleeping has been restless or disturbed some nights?

Insomnia Middle:

0 – No difficulty
1 – Complains of being restless and disturbed during the night
2 – Waking during the night – any getting out of bed (except to void) (22)

What time have you been waking up in the morning for the last time, this past week?

If early: Is that with an alarm clock, or do you just wake up yourself?

What time do you usually wake up (that is, before you got depressed)?

Insomnia Late:

0 – No difficulty
1 – Waking in early hours of
    morning but goes back to sleep
2 – Unable to fall asleep again if
    gets out of bed   (23)

How has your energy been this past week?

Have you been tired all the time?

This week, have you had any backaches, headaches, or muscles aches?

This week, have you felt any heaviness in your limbs, back or head?

Somatic Symptoms General:

0 – None
1 – Heaviness in limbs, back or
    head; backaches, headache,
    muscle aches; loss of
    energy and fatiguability
2 – Any clear-cut symptom   (24)

Have you been especially critical of yourself this past week, feeling you've done things wrong, or let others down?

If yes: What have your thoughts been?

Have you been feeling guilty about anything that you've done or not done?

Have you thought that you've brought (*this depression*) on yourself in some way?

Do you feel you're being punished by being sick?

Feelings of Guilt:

0 – Absent
1 – Self–reproach, feels he has let
    people down
2 – Ideas of guilt or rumination over
    past errors or sinful deeds
3 – Present illness is a punishment;
    delusions of guilt
4 – Hears accusatory or denunciatory
    voices and/or experiences
    threatening visual hallucinations   (25)

This past week, have you had any thoughts that life is not worth living, or that you'd be better off dead? What about having thoughts of hurting or even killing yourself?

If yes: What have you thought about? Have you actually done anything to hurt yourself?

Suicide:

0 – Absent
1 – Feels life is not worth living
2 – Wishes he were dead or any
    thoughts of possible death to self
3 – Suicidal ideas or gesture
4 – Attempts at suicide   (26)

Have you been feeling especially tense or irritable this past week?

Have you been worrying a lot about little unimportant things, things you wouldn't ordinarily worry about?
If yes: Like what, for example?

Anxiety Psychic:

0 – No difficulty
1 – Subjective tension and irritability
2 – Worrying about minor matters
3 – Apprehensive attitude apparent in
    face or speech
4 – Fears expressed without
    questioning   (27)

In this past week, have you had any physical symptoms that sometimes go along with being nervous, like (READ LIST, PAUSING AFTER EACH SYMPTOM FOR REPLY)?

How much have these things been bothering you this past week? (How bad have they gotten? How much of the time, or how often, have you had them?)

Note: Don't rate if clearly due to medication (e.g., dry mouth and imipramine)

In the last week, how much have your thoughts been focused on your physical health or how your body is working (compared to your normal thinking)?

Do you complain much about how you feel physically?

Have you found yourself asking for help with things you could really do yourself? *If yes*: Like what, for example? How often has that happened?

Rating Based on Observation

Rating Based on Observation During Interview

Anxiety Somatic (Physiological concomitants of anxiety, such as
GI   – Dry mouth, gas, indigestion, diarrhea, cramps, belching
C–V – Heart palpitations, headaches
Resp – Hyperventilating, sighing
Having to urinate frequently

Sweating:

0 – Absent
1 – Mild
2 – Moderate
3 – Severe
4 – Incapacitating   (28)

Hypochondriasis:

0 – Not present
1 – Self–absorption (bodily)
2 – Preoccupation with health
3 – Frequent complaints, requests for help, etc.
4 – Hypochondriacal delusions   (29)

Insight:

0 – Acknowledges being depressed and ill OR not currently depressed
1 – Acknowledges illness but attributes cause to bad food, climate, overwork, virus, need for rest, etc.
2 – Denies being ill at all   (30)

Retardation (slowness of thought and speech; impaired ability to concentrate; decreased motor activity):

0 – Normal speech and thought
1 – Slight retardation at interview
2 – Obvious retardation at interview
3 – Interview difficult
4 – Complete stupor   (31)

Rating Based on Observation
During Interview

Agitation:

0 – None
1 – Fidgetiness
2 – Playing with hands, hair, etc.
3 – Moving about, can't sit still
4 – Hand–wringing, nail–biting,
     hair-pulling, biting of lips   (32)

Total 17-item Hamilton Depression Score: (33-34)

This past week have you been feeling
better or worse at any particular
time of day – morning or evening?

Diurnal variation:

A. Note whether symptoms are worse
in morning or evening. If *no* diurnal
variation, mark none:

0 – No variation OR not currently
     depressed
1 – Worse in a.m.
2 – Worse in p.m.   (35)

If variation: How much worse do you
feel in the (*morning or evening*)?
If unsure: A little bit worse or a lot worse?

B. When present, mark the severity
of the variation:

0 – None
1 – Mild
2 – Severe   (36)

In the past week, have you ever
suddenly had the feeling that
everything is unreal, or you're in
a dream, or cut off from other
people in some strange way?
Any spacey feelings? *If yes:* How
bad has that been? How often this
week has that happened?

Depersonalization and derealization
(such as feelings of unreality and
nihilistic ideas):

0 – Absent
1 – Mild
2 – Moderate
3 – Severe
4 – Incapacitating   (37)

This past week, have you felt that
anyone was trying to give you a hard
time or hurt you?

If no: What about talking about you
behind your back?
If yes: Tell me about that.

Paranoid symptoms:

0 – None
1 – Suspicious
2 – Ideas of reference
3 – Delusions of reference and
     persecution   (38)

In the past week, have there been
things you've had to do over and
over again, like checking the locks
on the doors several times?

If yes: Can you give me an example?

Obsessional and compulsive symptoms:

0 – Absent
1 – Mild
2 – Severe   (39)

**Have you had any thoughts that
don't make any sense to you, but
that keep running over and over
in your mind?**

If yes: Can you give me an example?

Total 21-item Hamilton depression score: (40–41)
                                                                              60
                                                                          (79–80)0

The Hamilton Depression Scale and Its Alternatives: A Comparison of Their Reliability and Validity

W. MAIER[1]

1 Historical Developments

The efficacy of medical treatments is evidenced by a demonstrated reduction in the severity of the disorder being treated relative to a control condition. At the beginning of the era of psychopharmacology, in the late 1950s, neither a well-defined concept nor a well-defined measurement of the severity of depression, schizophrenia, or anxiety disorders were available. Consequently, it was difficult to compare groups of treated patients on the basis of treatment-specific rates of recovery. Hamilton was one of the first to recognize this lack and to create methods for standardizing the measurement of the effects of drugs across both patients and treatments. His idea was that a standardized measurement of the effects of drugs should be quantitative and specific for the various diagnostic categories.

In the absence of knowledge of the pathophysiology of psychiatric disorders, it was clear that the only possibility to describe the efficacy of drugs was in psychopathological terms. Psychiatric disorders such as depressive and anxiety disorders are complex conditions defined by the association of symptoms. Therefore two general measurements of the efficacy of drugs are possible: global assessments of change of the severity of a syndrome (using Likert scales) or counting and weighting symptoms associated with the disorder and summarizing these counts in a global score. Hamilton preferred the last-mentioned way and used the idea of rating scales developed in differential psychology to elaborate this concept. The advantage of rating scales was that powerful concepts such as reliability and validity and statistical techniques such as factor analysis had already been developed in psychology for evidencing that a particular scale is applicable and appropriate from a theoretical point of view. The Hamilton Depression (HAM-D) and the Hamilton Anxiety Rating Scales (HAM-A) were developed along these guidelines.

Three aspects inherent in the derivation of the Hamilton scales were subsequently criticized and motivated the development of alternative scales:

1. The assessment of severity using the Hamilton scales requires the diagnoses of depression (HAM-D) or anxiety neurosis (HAM-A); neither scale is intended for

---

[1] Department of Psychiatry, University of Mainz, Untere Zahlbacher Str. 8, 6500 Mainz 1, FRG

The Hamilton Scales
Editors: Per Bech and Alec Coppen
(Psychopharmacology Series 9)
© Springer-Verlag Berlin Heidelberg 1990

application in other disorders. However, this approach was criticized and a more comprehensive approach was recommended by Bech and Clemmesen (1983).

2. The symptoms included for the measurement of the severity of depression or anxiety are very heterogeneous ranging from core symptoms to symptoms only loosely associated with the disorder.

3. The validity of the Hamilton scales was mainly tested by using factor analysis and by correlations with global assessments measured by a single cross–sectional judgement. The sensitivity to change, which is the crucial criterion for testing the utility of measurements of drug effects, was originally not tested. Later on the sensitivity to change of the Hamilton scales (especially the HAM-D) was found to be imperfect (Montgomery and Asberg 1979).

These criticisms gave rise to developments resulting in new depression scales.

4. Bech et al. (1975) found the HAM-D to be unable to differentiate between moderate and severe levels of degree of depression; but they found a subscale of the HAM-D consisting of 6 core symptoms of depression (item no. 1 "depressed mood". no. 2 "guilt feelings", no. 7 "impaired work and social interest", no. 9 "retardation", no. 10 "psychic anxiety", no. 13 "somatic complaints"), discriminating moderate and severe states. The validity of this subscale was partly replicated by Maier and Philipp (1985a). The main difference between the two studies is that the item "somatic complaints" was substituted by the item "agitation" in the subscale derived by Maier and Philipp. Bech and Rafaelsen developed a new scale, the Bech-Rafaelsen Melancholia Scale (MES; Bech et al. 1986), extending the 6-item HAM-D subscale to an 11-item scale without extending the scope of symptoms included in the subscale. The scoring procedure was changed from the HAM-D: all items have five well-defined levels of severity and the meaning of the items as well as each level of severity are precisely characterized.

Moreover, Bech and Rafaelsen do not consider the MES to be an indicator only of severity in patients diagnosed as having depressive disorder; they also recommend using the MES items as aids for assessing diagnostic criteria and for determining the diagnoses of depression (Bech et al. 1983).

5. Montgomery and Asberg (1979) found the HAM-D to be insufficiently sensitive to change. They used the Clinical Psychiatric Rating Scale (CPRS), an inventory of items widely employed in Scandinavia and tapping a broad range of psychopathology, and identified those items showing maximal improvement during antidepressant treatment in depressed patients. They isolated 10 items and defined the Montgomery Asberg Depression scale (MADRS) by them. This scale mainly includes the core symptoms of depression. The items are graded on seven levels, four of them being well-defined and three in-between.

2 Yardsticks for Comparing Psychiatric Rating Scales

Two fundamental aspects need to be discriminated: reliability and validity. The major criterion for reliability is the test-retest condition describing the concordance rate of two ratings performed in two independent sessions in a limited period of time by independent raters (Williams 1988).

The major criteria of validity for rating scales are (a) content validity describing the adequacy of the content of the items intended to characterize the severity of a syndrome; (b) internal construct validity describing from a clinical point of view the homogeneity of the items and transferability of a scale across various samples and, from a statistical point of view, the statistical consistency (i.e., unidimensionality of the latent trait and the sufficiency of the total score); (c) well-defined external criteria of validity of rating scales are not available as no biological indicators of the severity of a psychiatric syndrome are known; and (d) the degree of psychosocial impairment may be a weak external criterion, but sometimes (e.g., in the HAM-D) it is considered to belong to the psychopathological indicators of severity, itself serving as an item of severity scales. Another alternative for testing the external validity of a scale is to use an independent global severity assessment by an expert taking all available data (including daily records and reports of the nurses as well as diaries by patients) as the yardstick. Spitzer (1983) called this procedure the LEAD (longitudinal expert assessment using all data) approach. Of course it is of only limited utility since the content of the criterion of validity is defined in psychopathological terms and is consequently not external to the measure to be validated.

Scales intended to measure the effects of drug should be primarily sensitive to change and should have a reasonable discriminatory power between inactive and active treatments. None of the scales mentioned above is perfect in all of these criteria — as will be demonstrated in the next sections.

A series of studies have compared the HAM-D with one of the alternative depression scales. Only a few reports have compared the three alternative depression scales mentioned above simultaneously using data from identical samples. The results of a comparison of these three depression rating scales are reviewed in the following sections. Additionally a fourth depression scale — a 5-item depression subscale derived from the HAM-D — is included in the comparison. This subscale comprises the items isolated by Bech et al. (1975) and are the most discriminative items mentioned above with the exception of the item "somatic complaints"; this particular item also did not belong to the homogeneous subscale derived by Maier and Philipp (1985a) using latent structure analysis.

We have reviewed the available evidence of the reliability and the validity of the HAM-D and other currently used depression scales referring additionally to our own comprehensive study (Maier et al. 1988a,b) based on data collected in the Department of Psychiatry, University of Mainz and on the literature.

2.1 Reliability (Table 1)

There are no major problems with the reliability of the total scores of the three depression scales being studied here, since each one is higher than .60. However, some items still lack sufficient reliability (Maier et al. 1988a; Rehm and O'Hara 1985; Cichetti and Prusoff 1983). Surprisingly, the 5-item version of the

Table 1. Test-Retest-Reliability between the total scores of two assessments by independent physicians within the same day before starting treatment and 3 weeks later ($n = 40$ inpatients with major depression)

Scales (total scores) tested for reliability	Intraclass coefficient	
	Before treatment	After treatment
HAM-D		
17 - item version	.72	.70
21 - item version	.70	.69
5 - item version	.69	.66
MADRS	.66	.82
MES	.79	.88

HAM-D yields a global score with sufficient reliability (intraclass coefficients higher than .60); the absolute values of the total score of the 5-item version are nearly as high as those for the longer versions with 17 and 21 items. This result is counter to what would have been expected because of a general theorem of psychomethrics that postulates that the higher the number of items in a homogeneous scale the higher the reliability. Generally, the *only* argument for a high number of items in homogeneous scales is the enhancement of reliability. But the HAM-D is not a homogeneous scale and therefore this psychometric theorem may not be valid.

2.2 Content Validity

The HAM-D (17- and 21-item versions) reflects the heterogeneity of depressive symptomatology by the heterogeneity of the contents of the items. A high load is given to somatic complaints (7 items). The 5-item version of the HAM-D ignores somatic complaints and focuses on psychosocial core symptoms of depression. The other two scales are also more homogeneous than the long versions of the HAM-D. The MES (11 items) stresses psychomotor disturbances by three items and the MADRS (10 items) stresses depressed mood and anhedonia by three items. Consequently, the three scales represent three very different concepts of the severity of depression. The three scales are intercorrelated sharing about 50% of variance (Pearson correlations between .60 and .80).

2.3 Internal Construct Validity (Table 2)

Internal construct validity requires the homogeneity and the transferability of the items and the sufficiency of the global score. A scale fulfilling these requirements refers to a well-defined latent variable, the global score is comparable across different samples of depressed patients metrically scaled on a dimension which is not observable directly and represents the variable to be measured (here: severity of depression). The global score summarizes all relevant information included in the items and is comparable across different samples on a one-dimensional metric scale. The Rasch model is the mathematical formula-

Table 2. Internal construct validity by Rasch model fitting of depression scales (in n = 130 inpatients with major depression)

Scale to be analysed	HAM-D (21 items)	HAM-D (17 items)	HAM-D (5 items)	MADRS	MES
Manner of partitioning:					
Chance	++	++	++	++	++
Age (Median)	++	++	++	++	++
Sex	++	++	++	++	++
Severity					
HAM-D (17 items) (Median)		−	−	+	− +
MADRS (Median)	−	−	++	+	++
MES (Median)	−	+	++	−	++
Diagnosis					
DSM-III-Major Depressive Episode with Melancholia	+	+	++	++	++
ICD-9 endogenous depression	−	−	++	++	++
Newcastle endogenous depression	+	+	+	+	+

+/++, Rasch model fitting ($P \geq 0.05$ / $P \geq 0.01$)
−, No Rasch model fitting ($P < .01$)

tion of these requirements. Scales fitting the Rasch model match these three requirements. Rasch model fitting is evidenced by the consistency of estimated item parameters between two disjunct subsamples. The total sample is subdivided using various clinically relevant criteria and the consistency of the estimates is tested for each of the criteria by dividing the sample into two subsamples. Table 2 summarizes our results from a sample with 130 acutely depressed inpatients. The long versions of the HAM-D (17- and 21-item versions) are at variance with the Rasch model. The short version of the HAM-D (5 items) as well as the MES are in agreement with the Rasch model. The MADRS yields inhomogeneous results, as was the case in a previous study (Maier and Philipp 1985b), as well. These results are in agreement with Bech et al. (1981) for the HAM-D and Allerup (1986) for the MADRS.

2.4 External Validity (Table 3)

In the absence of biological indicators of the severity of depression, the association between the global scores of the scales to be compared with other assessments of psychopathological and/or psychosocial variables may serve as the criterion of validity. A classical procedure is to use an independent global expert severity assessment involving all available data (LEAD approach) as the criterion of validity. All the rating scales being investigated here correlate highly with this yardstick. The figures for the HAM-D and the MADRS in Table 3 are similar to those reported by Kearns et al. (1982). The MES is superior to both

Table 3. External validity and sensitivity to change of three depression scales. Criterion of validity: independent assessment of global severity on a 10-point scale on baseline and endpoint and of change during 3 weeks treatment with tricyclics conducted by the treating physician using the LEAD approach (*n* = 42 psychiatric inpatients)

Rating scale[a]	Global assessment of severity		Global assessment of change
	Baseline (after 1 week washout)	Endpoint (after 3 weeks treatment)	
HAM-D (21 items)	.67	.74	.65
HAM-D (17 items)	.68	.74	.69
HAM-D (5 items)	.72	.77	.65
MADRS	.75	.81	.65
MES	.81	.80	.77

[a] The change on the scales, correlated with the global assessment of change in the third column, is represented by the residuals: the endpoint score is corrected for the baseline score

other scales in this respect (Table 3). The correlation coefficients of the 5-item version of the HAM-D are comparable to the correlation coefficients of the long versions of the HAM-D.

2.5 Sensitivity to Change (Table 3)

The optimal indicator for sensitivity to change is the ability of a scale to discriminate active from ineffective treatment in a reasonable number of patients randomized to either of the conditions. Preliminary evidence of sensitivity to change may be derived by correlating the change measured by the scales being studied here with the global assessment of change by an independent physician using all available information (LEAD approach). The change is measured by the residuals for each scale separately (observed score on endpoint minus score expected by the baseline score using a linear regression model). The MES is best under this criterion; all versions of the HAM-D also provide sufficient results (Table 3, last column).

Unfortunately there are no available data for a comparative assessment of the discriminative power of the scales investigated here with regard to active and ineffective treatment. Therefore, this crucial criterion of validity cannot be tested and all conclusions on the validity of the scales to be compared remain only preliminary.

3 Discussion

The HAM-D (17- and 21-item versions) and the two other currently used rating scales turned out to be reliable and valid instruments on their own, if the criterion of internal construct validity (introduced only recently to the field of scale analysis) is neglected. It is apparent by these results that the original versions of the HAM-D have stood the test of time.

The major flaw of the long versions of the HAM-D is the disagreement with the criterion of internal construct validity, tested by using the Rasch model. The consequence of the insufficient Rasch model fitting is that HAM-D scores cannot be compared across different samples or within a sample across different conditions (e.g., pre- and posttreatment). Especially the MES and to a lesser extent the MADRS are in this respect improvements on the original version of the HAM-D. But the 5-item version of the HAM-D also fits the requirements of both homogeneity and transferability. The missing validity of the original versions of the HAM-D is its heterogeneity of content. The data presented revealed no advantage being offered by the heterogeneity of the original version of the HAM-D. The long versions of the HAM-D are not more reliable than the 5-item version. Consequently, the original versions of the HAM-D are turning out to be rather ineconomic rating scales. However, an extension and more precise description of the core items of the HAM-D — as is proposed by the MES — might increase reliability and validity in comparison with the original HAM-D versions.

Drug studies traditionally refer to the HAM-D as the indicator for the efficacy of antidepressant treatment. However, a crucial condition for the comparison of different drug studies is the transferability of the indicator of efficacy. The HAM-D is not able to match this requirement. Each of the two more recently developed scales described here (especially the MES) provide a better basis for comparing different studies. Therefore, it is recommended that these scales be used in addition to the HAM-D. Alternatively, homogeneous subscales such as the 5-item version examined here may provide a transferable and valid measure of the effects of drugs.

Using the Hamilton scales as an item pool for selecting and redefining particular items for improved scales for rating depression, anxiety, and somatic complaints is probably the best way for the development of more valid measurements of the effects of drugs. The success of this procedure is elucidated by the validity of the 5-item version of the HAM-D which is clearly superior to the validity of the long versions of the HAM-D. Surely there is no need to develop new depression rating scales. What is needed are improvements of the depression scales already available in line with the criteria of validity.

References

Allerup P (1986) Statistical analysis of MADRS – a rating scale. Danish Institute for Educational Research, Copenhagen

Bech P, Clemmesen L (1983) The diagnosis of depression: 20 years later. Acta Pschiatr Scand [Suppl 310] 68:9–30

Bech P, Gram LF, Dein E, Jacobsen O, Vitger J, Bolwig TG (1975) Quantitative rating of depressive states. Correlation between clinical assessment, Beck's self-rating scale and Hamilton's objective rating scale. Acta Psychiatr Scand 51:161–170

Bech P, Allerup P, Gram L, Reisby N, Rosenberg R, Jacobsen D, Nagy A (1981) The Hamilton rating scale: evaluation of objectivity using logistic models. Acta Psychiatr Scand 63:290–299

Bech P, Gjerris A, Andersen J, Bøjholm S, Kramp P, Bolwig TG, Kastrup M, Clemmesen L, Rafaelsen OJ (1983) The melancholia scale and the Newcastle scales. Item-combinations and inter-observer reliability. Br J Psychiatry 143:58–63

Bech P, Kastrup M, Rafaelsen OJ (1986) Mini-compendium of rating scales for anxiety, depression, mania, schizophrenia with corresponding DSM-III syndromes. Acta Psychiatr Scand [Suppl 326] 73:1–39

Cichetti DV, Prusoff BA (1983) Reliability of depression and associated clinical symptoms. Arch Gen Psychiatry 40:987–990

Hamilton M (1960) A rating scale for depression. J Neurol Neurosurg Psychiatry 23:56–62

Hamilton M (1967) Development of a rating scale for primary depressive illness. Br J Soc Clin Psychol 6:276–296

Kearns NP, Cruikshank CA, McGuigan K, Rilag SA, Shaw SP, Snaith RP (1982) A comparison of depression rating scales. Br J Psychiatry 141:45–49

Maier W, Philipp M (1985a) Improving the assessment of severity of depressive states: a reduction of the Hamilton depression scale. Pharmacopsychiatry 18:114–115

Maier W, Philipp M (1985b) Comparative analysis of observer depression scales. Acta Psychiatr Scand 72:239–245

Maier W, Philipp M, Heuser I, Schlegel S, Buller R, Wetzel H (1988) Improving depression severity assessment. I. Reliability, internal validity and sensitivity to change of three observer depression scales. J Psychiatr Res 22:3–12

Maier W, Heuser I, Philipp M, Frommberger U, Demuth W (1988) Improving depression severity assessment. II. Content, concurrent and external validity of three observer depression scales. J Psychiatr Res 22:13–19

Montgomery SA, Asberg M (1979) A new depression scale designed to be sensitive to change. Br J Psychiatry 134:382–389

Rehm L, O'Hara MW (1985) Item characteristics of the Hamilton rating scale for depression. J Psychiatr Res 19:31–42

Roth M, Gurney C, Mountjoy CQ (1983) The Newcastle rating scales for depression. Acta Psychiatr Scand [Suppl 310] 68: 42–54

Spitzer RL (1983) Psychiatric Diagnosis: Are clinicians still necessary? Compr Psychiatry 24:399-411

Williams JBW (1988) A structured interview guide for the Hamilton depression rating scale. Arch Gen Psychiatry 45:742–747

Psychometric Developments of the Hamilton Scales: The Spectrum of Depression, Dysthymia, and Anxiety

P. BECH[1]

1 Psychometric Methods

The history of mental rating scales begins with the intelligence scales developed by Binet (1903). As stated by Terman and Merrill (1957): "...the Binet type of scales has no serious rival. It is not merely an intelligence test; it is a method of standardized interview...." In the field of depression and anxiety this statement is valid for the Hamilton scales. They are not merely scales. They are information collected by a standardized interview, and both Hamilton scales have no serious rivals as they cover the universe of items within clinical depression and anxiety.

Since the introduction of the Binet scales, psychometric methods have been developed for defining the dimension of intelligence. The two most useful methods in this respect have been factor analysis (Spearman 1904; Guildford 1936) and latent structure analysis (Guttman 1950; Rasch 1960). Both psychometric methods have been applied to the Hamilton scales.

2 Factor Analysis of the Hamilton Depression Scale (HAM-D)

When Hamilton (1960) published his depression scale he used factor analysis to define the dimension of severity of depressive states. However, no general factor was found. In his second study with the HAM-D a general factor of severity was found (Hamilton 1967). As pointed out by Hamilton himself (Hamilton 1986) the reason for this discrepancy between the two studies was that the heterogeneity of the patients regarding severity of depression was larger in the second than in the first study. It is one of the drawbacks of the factor analytic method, that it is sensitive to the distribution of the population under investigation. When summarizing the many studies that have been carried out on the HAM-D with factor analysis, Hamilton (1986) has stated that most investigators would accept two factors in the scale, a general factor of severity and a second for anxious-agitated depression.

[1] Frederiksborg General Hospital, Department of Psychiatry, 48 Dyrehavevej, 3400 Hillerød, Denmark

The Hamilton Scales
Editors: Per Bech and Alec Coppen
(Psychopharmacology Series 9)
© Springer-Verlag Berlin Heidelberg 1990

Table 1. Classification of depression by symptoms

ICD-10	DSM-III-R	MES
Classical textbook classification	Prototypic classification	Latent structure analysis
	1 Depressed mood	1 Work and interests
Lowering mood	2 Markedly diminished interest	2 Lowered mood
Reduction of energy and activity	3 Significant weight loss or weight gain	3 Sleep disturbances
Reduction of enjoyment and interest	4 Insomnia or hypersomnia	4 Anxiety
Impaired concentration	5 Psychomotor agitation or retardation	5 Emotional retardation
Marked tiredness	6 Fatigue or loss of energy	6 Intellectual retardation
Disturbed sleep	7 Feelings of worthlessness or excessive guilt	7 Tiredness and pain
Diminished appetite	8 Diminished ability to concentrate	8 Guilt feelings
Reduced self-esteem	9 Recurrent thoughts of death	9 Decreased verbal activity
Guilt feelings		10 Suicidal thoughts
Suicidal thoughts		11 Decreased motor activity

3 Latent Structure Analysis of the HAM-D Scale

Among the first to develop an alternative psychometric method to factor analysis within intelligence tests was Guttman (1950). He emphasized that the Binet scaling principle should be analysed for its ability to separate the brighter person from the duller. Guttman's hierarchical construct of intelligence implied that the items of an intelligence scale should have a rank order of difficulty; i.e., the least difficult items are listed first, the moderately difficult items in the middle, and the most difficult items are listed in the end. As the brighter person is able to respond adequately to most of the items while the duller person only is able to respond adequately to the less difficult items, the total score of adequate items response is a sufficient statistic of the dimension of intelligence. Hamilton (1976) made an attempt to analyse his depression scale using the Guttman scalogram principle but focussed only on one item, depressed mood.

We used the latent structure analysis developed by Rasch (1960) in validating the HAM-D (Bech et al. 1981). This Rasch method is a further construct of the Guttman scalogram analysis taking probabilistic theories of errors of measurement into account. We found that the structure of severity of depressive states in the HAM-D could be sufficiently defined by six items (indicated by the letters a to f in Table 2). On the basis of these six HAM-D items we (Bech and Rafaelsen 1980) developed the Melancholia Scale (MES) which has a hierarchical structure in the sense of Guttman as shown in Table 1. Patients with minor depression or dysthymia scored on the first items including anxiety and

Table 2. Universe of items and their combinations

Item	HAM-D (17)	MES (11)	HAM-A (8 + 6)	CIS	MADRS Index
Depressed mood	a ☐	☐	☐	☐	x3
Guilt	b ☐	☐			x1.5
Suicide	☐	☐			x1.5
Initial	☐				
Middle	☐				
Late	☐				
Work	c ☐	☐			x1.5
Retardation (motor)	d ☐				
Agitation (motor)	☐		☐		
Anxiety (psychic)	e ☐	☐	☐	☐	x1.5
Anxiety (somatic)	☐		☐ (6)	☐	
Gastrointestinal	☐				
Somatic general	f ☐				
Sex	☐				
Hypochondriasis	☐				
Loss of insight	☐				
Weight	☐				
Insomnia (general)		☐	☐	☐	x1.5
Motor retardation		☐			
Verbal retardation		☐			
Intellectual retardation		☐	☐		x1.5
Emotional retardation		☐			x1.5
Tiredness and pains		☐	☐	☐	
Tension (inner)			☐	☐	
Phobia			☐		

tiredness, while patients with major depression also scored on items of guilt, motor activity, and suicidal thoughts (Table 1). This rank order of symptoms is in accordance with Hamilton's last paper, released posthumously, in which Hamilton emphasizes that anxiety is an important symptom in depression (Hamilton 1989).

Our results with the MES have been confirmed in other studies with the scale on the basis of Rasch analysis (e.g., Maier and Philipp 1985; Maier et al. 1988a; Chambon et al. 1990).

4 Consequences of the Psychometric Studies with the HAM-D Scale

Table 1 shows the psychometric development in the classification of depression from the ICD system (e.g., ICD-10), the DSM-III-R system, and the MES modification of the HAM-D.

The ICD system is based on the classical textbook classification where no structure is needed. The DSM-III-R is based on the prototype algorithm meaning that the symptoms indicated in Table 1 have a higher mutual correlation than they do with other symptoms in the DSM-III-R. This prototypic approach (e.g., Cantor et al. 1980) is identical with the principle of factors in factor analysis. The latent structure analysis is an approach identical to the concept of transparency used by Feinstein (1987) which refers to the ability to see through each level of total scores of a rating scale to determine what it contains. As indicated in Table 1 a total MES score of 0 to 5 means no depression; a score of 6 to 14 means minor depression or dysthymia; and a score of 15 or more means major depression.

The dimension of severity of depression in the HAM-D as defined by Rasch analysis has been supported by external validity studies. It correlated with the global assessment performed by experienced psychiatrists (Bech et al. 1975). Pretreatment classification of patients with panic disorder into no, minor, and major depression had predictive validity concerning response to imipramine versus placebo (Bech et al., in preparation), as no difference was seen in patients without depression while imipramine was superior in depressed patients.

When used as measure of outcome of antidepressive treatment a negative correlation between the HAM-D subscale and plasma levels of clomipramine was found posttreatmently (Bech 1984). Furthermore, Rosenberg et al. (1988) have demonstrated that the total score of the HAM-D subscale correlated significantly with cerebral blood flow values pretreatmently, while such an association was not found using the 17-item HAM-D total scores or the items individually.

Finally, it has been shown that placebo-active drug differences in clinical trials with antidepressants are more pronounced when using the HAM-D subscale than the 17-item HAM-D (Bech 1989).

Table 2 shows the universe of items of the HAM-D and MES. To our knowledge rating scales for depression currently in use in psychotherapy, social psychiatry, or epidemiological psychiatry have no items which cannot be found in the HAM-D/MES universe. One of the most frequently used self-rating scales in epidemiological psychiatry, the General Health Questionnaire (Goldberg 1972) can be considered to be a patient-rated version of the MES (Bech 1987). The scale measuring minor psychiatric cases in the setting of general practice (Clinical Interview Schedule, CIS; Goldberg and Huxley 1980) is also covered by the universe of items in Table 2.

A scale developed to be sensitive to change during psychopharmacological treatment by Montgomery and Åsberg (1979), the Montgomery-Åsberg Depression Rating Scale (MADRS), is included in the HAM-D/MES universe as well (Table 2). This scale seems less sensitive to change during treatment compared with the MES (Maier et al. 1988a). Using 50% reduction of pretreatment score the MADRS was found less sensitive than the HAM-D (Bech 1989). Furthermore, Maier (1987, personal communication) has correlated the HAM-D/MES version of MADRS (Table 2) with the original MADRS version in a study including 118 depressed patients. A correlation coefficient of 0.91 was obtained. The intercept of the regression line was 1.6 with a slope of 0.9. In other words, a score of 10 on the MADRS corresponds to 10.6 on the HAM-D/MES version; a score of 20 on MADRS corresponds to 19.6 on the HAM-D/MES version.

Likewise, we have found that a score of 15 or more on the MES corresponds to a major depression on DSM-III (Bech et al. 1983). The group of items defining the DSM-III concept of dysthymia is also included the universe of items in Table 2.

The universe of items in Table 2 has, however, no coverage of items for the depressive triade of negative self-evaluation of past, present, and future. The first scale that covered these items was the Wechsler Scale (1963). This scale has, however, not been frequently used in clinical research.

5 Factor Analysis of the Hamilton Anxiety Scale (HAM-A)

In his first study with this scale Hamilton (1959) found a general factor as the first factor and a bipolar factor as the second (psychic versus somatic anxiety). In his second study these findings were confirmed (Hamilton 1969). In both studies Hamilton investigated patients with anxiety neuroses. We have recently, in a population of patients with panic disorders (Bech et al., in preparation), replicated the findings of Hamilton.

6 Latent Structure Analysis of the HAM-A Scale

When using the HAM-A outside its original scope (anxiety neurosis) we found that the factor of psychic anxiety was most relevant in depressive illness (Gjerris et al. 1983). In patients evaluated before cardiac bypass surgery we found (Bech et al. 1984) a high correlation between HAM-A and MES ($R=0.91$). In the latter study only 3% had a major depression while 63% had a minor depression. In a study using Rasch analysis, Maier et al. (1988b) found that the psychic anxiety factor of HAM-A fulfilled the Rasch criteria in contrast to the total HAM-A or the somatic anxiety factor. This finding is in harmony with a Rasch analysis carried out in patients with panic disorders (Bech et al., in preparation).

7 The Universe of HAM-D, MES, and HAM-A

Table 2 shows the relevant items of the HAM-A in relation to the HAM-D/ MES universe. Of these items depressed mood, psychic anxiety, insomnia in general, and intellectual retardation are identical to the corresponding MES items that cover minor depression. The original HAM-D item of general muscular symptoms corresponds to the MES item of tiredness and pains. The original HAM-A item of behaviour at interview corresponds to the HAM-D item of agitation, but it seems that this item should not be included in the dimension of severity (Bech et al., in preparation). The HAM-D item of somatic anxiety can be considered to be a general item of autonomic hyperactivity which might be of importance in describing the minor degrees of depression. Two important HAM-A items, tension and phobia, should be included to cover the whole dimension of anxiety. In conclusion, therefore, we have included tension and phobia in the HAM-D/MES universe to cover also the HAM-A. The eight HAM-A items should be further analysed by Rasch models to test whether they describe mild degrees of minor depression.

8 Test of Time of the Hamilton Scales

It has often been stated that it was the introduction of antidepressants in the years before the publication of the Hamilton rating scales that induced the need for scales measuring outcome of treatment. However, it is often overlooked that the Hamilton scales themselves have, if properly administered, a "therapeutic" effect. Before the introduction of antidepressants, Skottowe (1953) in his integrated textbook of psychiatry made the following observation: "The initial psychiatric interview is always important, but in no group of illnesses is it of greater importance as a first step in treatment than it is in the depressions. The gentle elucidation of *all* the symptoms is of the highest importance. Let the patient see that the doctor is thoroughly familiar with the kind of illness that confronts him; he knows the kind of feelings and thoughts that it brings to the patient. This in itself is a most reassuring step." The universe of items on the Hamilton scales (Table 2) will guide the doctor, thereby giving the patient relief as stated by Skottowe.

In the historical validation it is interesting to note that in the controlled clinical trials on antidepressants, symptom-rating scales have outdated psychological tests (Quality Assurance Project 1983). In an overview of antidepressant drug trials published between 1964 and 1986 in elderly depressed patients, Gerson et al. (1988) have shown that the HAM-D made other contemporary scales obsolete by around 1976.

When making a metaanalytic review of antidepressant drugs (Bech 1988), it became clear that there are many different versions of the HAM-D. The original item definitions were often inadequate and included versions separating males and females which, of course, is due to historical reasons. It seems that the most frequently used versions of the Hamilton scales are those published by Guy (1976), often referred to as the NIMH versions. However, Hamilton never accepted these versions which he considered as checklist scales (Hamilton 1986).

The operational criteria we recently have published were developed in collaboration with Hamilton (Bech et al. 1986).

9 Conclusion

The universe of items covered by the HAM-D and HAM-A scales is an important guide for the doctor making the initial psychiatric interview with the anxious or depressed patient. Like the Binet scales for measuring intelligence the Hamilton scales can be considered as a method of standardizing a clinical interview.

The psychometric methods of factor analysis and latent structure analysis have illustrated the complementary problem of the primary (general) dimension of depression or anxiety versus the many second order dimensions. The results with the HAM-D have shown that a general dimension of severity has been isolated, the melancholia subscale, which has led to the MES to be considered as a one-dimensional scale.

Various validity studies have confirmed this general dimension of severity of depression, which, inter alia, is relevant when comparing the relative potency of antidepressant drugs. Among the second order dimensions the anxiety factor and the sleep factor have been most important when describing the profile of antidepressants. In the HAM-A scale there are two main factors of which the psychic anxiety factor includes items relevant for mild depression or dysthymia.

Both the anxiety scale and the depression scale were released by Hamilton with rather insufficient operational definitions which have resulted in many attempts to make revised item definitions. It is important to reach a consensus regarding this aspect of the Hamilton scales. In a chapter on Binet to be found in the monograph of scientific psychology, Miller (1964) has stated that: "...the vein that Binet opened up is still being mined today — and still yields ore of the highest grade...." This statement is valid for Max Hamilton, as well, indicated in this psychometric overview of his rating scales.

References

Bech P (1984) The instrumental use of rating scales for depression. Pharmacopsychiatry 17:22–28

Bech P (1987) Quality of life in psychosomatic research. Psychopathology 20:169–179

Bech P (1988) A review of the antidepressants properties of serotonin reuptake inhibitors. In: Gastpar M, Wakelin J (eds) Advances in biological psychiatry. Karger, Basel, pp 58–69

Bech P (1989) Clinical effects of selective serotonin reuptake inhibitors. In: Dahl SG, Gram LF (eds) Clinical pharmacology in psychiatry. Springer, Berlin Heidelberg New York Tokyo, pp 81–93

Bech P, Rafaelsen OJ (1980) The use of rating scales exemplified by a comparison of the Hamilton and the Bech-Rafaelsen melancholia scale. Acta Psychiatr Scand [Suppl 285] 62:128–131

Bech P, Gram LF, Dein E, Jacobsen O, Vitger J, Bolwig TG (1975) Quantitative rating of depressive states. Acta Psychiatr Scand 51:161–170

Bech P, Allerup P, Gram LF, Reisby N, Rosenberg R, Jacobsen O, Nagy A (1981) The Hamilton depression scale. Evaluation of objectivity using logistic models. Acta Psychiatr Scand 63:290–299

Bech P, Gjerris A, Andersen J (1983) The melancholia rating scale and the Newcastle scales. Br J Psychiatry 143:58–63

Bech P, Allerup P, Reisby N, Gram LF (1984) Assessment of symptom change from improvement curves on the Hamilton depression scale in trials with antidepressants. Psychopharmacology (Berlin) 84:276–281

Bech P, Kastrup M, Rafaelsen OJ, (1986) Mini-compendium of rating scales for states of anxiety, depression, mania, schizophrenia with corresponding DSM-III syndromes. Acta Psychiatr Scand [Suppl 326] 73:1–37

Binet A (1903) L'étude expérimentale de l'intelligence. Schleicher, Paris

Cantor N, Smith EE, French RS, Mezzich J (1980) Psychiatric diagnoses as prototype categorization. J Abnorm Psychol 89:181–193

Chambon O, Cialdella P, Kiss L, Poncet F (1990) Study of the unidimensionality of the Bech-Rafaelsen melancholia scale using Rasch analysis in a French sample of major depressive disorders. Pharmacopsychiatry (in press)

Feintein AR (1987) Clinimetrics. Yale University Press, New Haven

Gerson SC, Plotkin DA, Jarvik LF (1988) Antidepressant drug studies, 1964 to 1986: empirical evidence for aging patients. J Clin Psychopharmacol 8:311–322

Gjerris A, Bech P, Bøjholm S (1983) The Hamilton anxiety scale. J Affective Disord 5:163–170

Goldberg D (1972) The detection of psychiatric illness by questionnaire. Oxford University Press, Oxford

Goldberg D, Huxley P (1980) Mental illness in the community. Tavistock, London

Guildford JP (1936) Psychometric methods. McGraw-Hill, New York

Guttman L (1950) The basis for scalogram analysis. In: Stouffer SA, Guttman L, Suchman EA, Lazarsfeld PF, Starr SS, Clausen JA (eds) Measurement and prediction. Princeton University Press, Princeton, pp 60–90

Guy W (1976) Early clinical drug evaluation (ECDEU) assessment manual for psychopharmacology. National Institute of Mental Health, Rockville, USA, Publication no. 76–338

Hamilton M (1959) The assessment of anxiety states by rating. Br J Med Psychol 32:50–55

Hamilton M (1960) A rating scale for depression. J Neurol Neurosurg Psychiatry 23:56–62

Hamilton M (1967) Development of a rating scale for primary depressive illness. Br J Soc Clin Psychol 6:278–296

Hamilton M (1969) Diagnosis and rating of anxiety. Br J Psychiatry [Spec Publ] 3:76–79

Hamilton M (1976) Clinical evaluation of depressions: clinical criteria and rating scales, including a Guttman scale. In: Gallant DM, Simpson GM (eds) Depression: behavioral, biochemical, diagnostic and treatment concept. Spectrum, New York, pp 155–179

Hamilton M (1986) The Hamilton rating scale for depression. In: Sartorius N, Ban T (eds) Assessment of depression. Springer, Berlin Heidelberg New York, pp 143–152

Hamilton M (1989) Frequency of symptoms in melancholia (depressive illness). Br J Psychiatry 154:201–206

Maier W, Philipp M (1985) Comparative analysis of observer depression scales. Acta Psychiatr Scand 72:230–245

Maier W, Philipp M, Heuser I, Schlegel S, Buller R, Wetzel H (1988a) Improving depression severity assessment. Reliability, internal validity and sensitivity to change of three observer depression scales. J Psychiatr Res 22:3–12

Maier W, Buller R, Philipp M, Heuser I (1988b) The Hamilton anxiety scale. Reliability, validity and sensitivity to change in anxiety and depressive disorders, J Affective Disord 14:61–68

Miller GA (1964) Psychology: the science of mental life. Hutchinson, London

Montgomery SA, Asberg M (1979) A new depression scale designed to be sensitive to change. Br J Psychiatry 111:240–242

Quality Assurance Project (1983) A treatment outline for depressive disorders. Aust N Z J Psychiatry 17:129–146

Rasch G (1960) Probabilistic models for some intelligence and attainment tests. Danish Institute for Educational Research, Copenhagen

Rosenberg R, Vorstrup S, Andersen A, Bolwig TB (1988) Effect of ECT on cerebral blood flow in melancholia assessed with SPECT. Convulsive Ther 4:62–73

Skottowe I (1953) Clinical psychiatry. Eyre and Spottiswoode, London

Spearman C (1904) General intelligence: objectively determined and measured. Am J Psychol 15:201–293

Terman CM, Merrill MA (1957) Measuring intelligence. Houghton Mifflin, New York

Wechsler H, Grosser GH, Busfield BL (1963) The depression rating scale. A quantitative approach to the assessment of depressive symptomatology. Arch Gen Psychiatry 9:334–343

The Hamilton Depression Scale and the Numerical Description of the Symptoms of Depression*

G.E. Berrios[1] and A. Bulbena-Villarasa[2]

1 Introduction

Psychiatric symptoms can be pictured in words or numbers (Berrios 1984). In either case information is gathered for clinical or research purposes. Ideally, the process ought to be fully reversible, that is, data stores ought to be able to release information at any time without distortion or fuss. The grammar governing the conversion of a symptom into a scale item, however, has not yet been fully decoded (Robins 1989). Psychiatric scales are devices to gather and store information. Although a great deal is known about their construction and formal operation (Brown and Thomson 1925; Cronbach et al. 1972; Ghiselli et al. 1981), knowledge on their information-carrying properties is still elementary.

Conventionally, the *item* has been considered as the smallest information-carrying unit, and since the 1930s, much research has been done on its mathematical properties (Osterlind 1983). For example, item values can be added and this curious feature is considered by some as a justification to use global scores as continuous magnitudes. More to the point, however, items are not equal in their information-carrying capacity. So, scales usually show regions of high information density which on analysis may give rise to "subscales" or "factors". Apart from reflecting differences between items, this uneven distribution of information may also reflect the very nature of the disease the scale is endeavouring to quantify.

But in addition to the information stored in items and in item clusters, information related to general endorsement patterns also becomes trapped in the total numerical matrix of the scale. For example, in the Hamilton Depression Rating Scale (HAM-D; Hamilton 1960), at least three information loci may be available: the individual item (e.g. depression or guilt or early awakening); item arrays or subscales (e.g. symptoms representing an "endogenous" factor); and the overall numerical patterns. It is likely that each locus requires a different

* This paper is based on a lecture given by GEB on 30th May 1989 at Downing College, Cambridge, and is dedicated to the memory of Max Hamilton under whose tutorage he regained his earlier interest in mathematics.
[1] Department of Psychiatry, University of Cambridge, Addenbrooke's Hospital (Level 4), Hills Road, Cambridge CB2 2QQ, UK
[2] Departamento de Neurociencias, Universidad del País Vasco, Lejona, Vizcaya, Spain

The Hamilton Scales
Editors: Per Bech and Alec Coppen
(Psychopharmacology Series 9)
© Springer-Verlag Berlin Heidelberg 1990

information-extracting methodology. Calculation of global scores and analyses of subscales are adequate for the first two; methods for squeezing information from the number matrix, however, are not yet fully available. Consequently, it is plausible to suggest that information remains unused in the bowels of all psychiatric scales.

Only an efficient extraction of this information from all three loci will allow for adequate comparisons between, say, the HAM-D and other instruments sharing a similar clinical territory such as the Beck, Zung, or Bech. Differences between these scales may be traced back to methods of assessment or item choice (Paykel and Norton 1986; Bech 1981; Bech et al 1975; 1979).

This chapter will illustrate some of these problems by giving a brief account of the history and evolution of the HAM-D, and in particular of Hamilton's private views on the information-carrying characteristics of his scale. It will also report some data based on the analysis of 1204 Spanish cases suffering from affective disorder: 430 with DSM-III major depression and 774 with DSM-III dysthymic disorder (APA 1980).

2 The Hamilton Depression Scale

Although Hamilton had been toying with the idea at least since 1956, the first version of his depression scale was only published in 1960 (Hamilton 1959; 1960; 1983). He devised the scale "for use only on patients already diagnosed as suffering from affective disorder of depressive type". It was to be used "for quantifying the results of an interview" (Hamilton 1960, p.56). These two points are important: the HAM-D was not meant to be a diagnostic scale but to measure what Hamilton called years later "the burden of disease"; it was also meant to capture *state* rather than *trait* features, that is phenomena susceptible to change. Hence, its sources of information included not only direct clinical assessment but also anyone who knew the patient. The most important conclusion to be drawn from this is that since it was not a diagnostic scale, there was no reason to include all, or even the most important symptoms of depression. (Important, that is, in terms of any putative aetiological view.) This is the reason why Hamilton (1965) was also sceptical as to whether the HAM-D could be used in clinical prediction.

Hamilton chose his items in terms of symptom frequency, facility for rating, and susceptibility to change; 21 items were included but only 17 considered for the core of the scale; the other 4 were to be rated separately (either because they were not considered as part of the disease or did not reflect severity, or because they were infrequent). Some items were to be rated on a 3-, and others on a 5-point scale. Although these ratings constitute de facto weightings, Hamilton did not mean them to be so. The 3-point scale was chosen when "quantification of the variable was either difficult or impossible". Originally, the scale was meant to be rated by two raters and their ratings added up. If only one rater was utilized the score had to be doubled.

The original factor analysis was carried out on data from 49 males and regression equations were calculated from 64 patients (Hamilton 1960). Since the original analysis did not extract any factors resembling the clinical syndromes, Hamilton suggested that discriminant function analysis might be used instead. None was carried out in the original paper.

Perusal of his early work is important for it includes Hamilton's views on factor analysis. For example, and very much in Cyril Burt's tradition, he wrote that "factor analysis, except for the method of principal component with full variance, actually loses information..." (Hamilton 1959, p. 52). This is only true in a technical sense. It is now known that alternative algorithms to principal component analysis, such as factor analysis, do not make use of all the variance contained in the matrix and hence can be said to "lose" information. But this selectivity confers an advantage: extracted factors are cleaner, more circumscribed, and hence easier to interpret (Comrey 1973; Tinsley and Tinsley 1987).

As to the origin or the information stored in the scale, Hamilton held a "realistic" view, i.e., he believed that during rating information was directly transferred from the behavioural phenomenon to the item. He also believed that the fact that his scale relied on multiple information sources constituted an advantage over the self-administered scales.

With regard to the meaning or conceptual status of the factors themselves, Hamilton followed the meandering path traced by his teacher, Cyril Burt, who, as it is well known, vascillated between considering factors as mathematical abstractions and as true representations of brain sites (Burt 1940). Burt's hesitations are understandable both in terms of his personality and professional work: after all he was interested in the analysis of abstract concepts such as intelligence or delinquent behaviour (Hearnshaw 1979).

Clinicians such as Hamilton, however, had a different view of the way in which the symptoms of depression related to the brain. Although his earliest views on depression antedate the neurochemical hypotheses, he upheld an organic view of endogenous depression throughout. But, like many of his generation, he also shared in the ante-bellum holism of Adolf Meyer. So, it was difficult for him to accept that factor analysis could ever help to test hypotheses with regards to the cerebral localization of depression (Hamilton 1967a, pp. 286-87). This resistance was compounded by the fact that he conceived of factors as orthogonal entities, that is, as representing uncorrelated sources of variance. (Indeed, Hamilton had been an orthogonalist even before Kaiser started publishing his work; see Hamilton (1960). So, it must have been intellectually repugnant to him to consider depressive illness as a mere admixture of symptom clusters originating in unrelated brain sites.

Again, under the influence of the British factorists (Spearman 1932; Burt 1940; Thomson 1950), Hamilton showed little interested in oblique rotations (Thurstone 1947) although he knew about them (Hamilton 1960, p.59). This was a pity for such a useful method might have allowed him to reconcile his clinical hunch with the structure of the scale, i.e. to show that the factors themselves (or their related brain sites) did indeed covary. It can be safely said that Hamilton utilized factor analysis more as a tool to establish the structure of the scale than as a technique to elucidate the biology and classification of depression. To be fair to him, however, these usages only came later. During the period when Hamilton was interested in factor analysis, the work of the second generation of factor analysts had not yet been appeared (Comrey 1973; Lawley and Maxwell 1963; Kim and Mueller 1978a,b). So, the useful distinction between the conceptual, statistical and mathematical aspects of factor analysis was not yet available.

The recent shift towards brain localization and modularity of brain functions (Fodor 1983; Shallice 1988) has, once again, posed the question of symptom localization in mental illness. Once again factor analysis may be considered as potentially useful in this regard, particularly because of current awareness of its complexities and limitations. For example, it can identify orthogonal factors in neuropsychiatric research where the idea of independently affected brain sites is more acceptable (Politynska et al. 1990; Dening and Berrios 1989).

In 1967 Hamilton published a further account of his scale based this time on 152 men and 120 women, and also a paper (written 3 years earlier), on the application of Ahmavaara's method for goodness-of-fit between homologous factors obtained from different samples from the same putative population (Hamilton 1967b). Since then, the number-crunching involved in factor analysis has been alleviated by the availability of microcomputers. This has led to the publication of a large number of papers applying factor analysis to the Hamilton scale (Hedlund and Vieweg 1979; O'Brien and Glaudin 1988). This work has been addressed to seven issues: scale construction, summary of information, classifications, item analysis, factorial structure, diagnostic function, and search for loci of change.

This chapter reports data relevant to only three of these topics: (a) item analysis and the effect on endorsement patterns of sex, age, and national differences; (b) DSM III diagnoses and its association with HAM-D; and (c) the factorial structure of HAM-D.

3 Subjects and Methods

The data to be produced are based on as sample of 1204 Spanish subjects evaluated three times. The HAM-D has been validated in Castilian (Ramos and Cordero 1986a,b). Theoretical worries that Spanish depressives might show a high endorsement of somatic symptoms have proven unfounded (Ramos and Cordero 1987a,b). Factorial studies show that the structure of the scale in Spanish samples does not differ significantly from that in other countries (Cordero and Ramos 1986).

The original 21-item version of the scale was used, and only 17 items included in the analysis. Patients were first diagnosed according to DSM-III (APA 1980) criteria for either major depression or dysthymia and then assessed by means of the HAM-D on days 0, 15 and 42. Age, sex, weight, and other clinical data were also collected and global clinical evaluations of severity of

Table 1. The Spanish Sample. Three HAM-D 17-items ratings per patient (on days 0, 15, and 42)

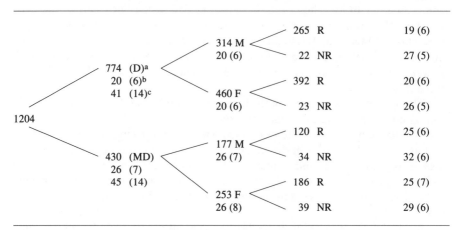

a Dsythymia (D), and major depression (MD) (DSM-III)
b HAM-D score = mean (SD) at day 0
c Age = mean (SD)
R, responder; NR, nonresponder (GAS+HAM-D)
(addition of R + NR shows missing data: drop-outs)

disease recorded by the clinicians in charge. The occasion for the collection of this large sample was the multicentre Spanish trial of Minaprine. Statistical analysis was carried out in Cambridge, UK, in an IBM-AT PC; version 3 of the SPSS PC+ package was used throughout.

4 Results

4.1 General

Table 1 shows the composition of the sample. There were 774 cases diagnosed as DSM-III dysthymia (DD) and 430 as DSM-III major depression (MD). The mean Hamilton scores for the dysthymics was 20 with a standard deviation of 6; of the major depressives 26, with a standard deviation of 7. The mean age for the two diagnostic groups was 41 and 45 years, respectively. Table 1 also shows the diagnostic groups split by gender. In the dysthymic group there were 314 males and 460 females; in the major depression 177 males and 253 females. Mean and standard deviation of global Hamilton score are included for the four subgroups. Finally, proportions of responders and nonresponders and their initial global scores and SD (in brackets) are shown. Distributions for global scores, "improvement" scores (obtained by subtracting the third from the first Hamilton), and subject's age were not skewed.

Table 2. Major depression. Differences in HAM-D ratings according to sex ($n=430$)

	Male n=77		Female n=253		Two-tailed t-test
1. Depressed mood	3.	(.9) [a]	3.1	(.9)	NS
2. Guilt	1.6	(1)	1.5	(1)	NS
3. Suicide	1.	(.9)	1.2	(1)	.05
4. Insomnia, initial	1.3	(.8)	1.3	(.7)	NS
5. Insomnia, middle	.9	(.8)	.9	(.7)	NS
6. Insomnia, delayed	1.2	(.8)	1.1	(.8)	NS
7. Work and interest	3.0	(.9)	2.7	(.9)	.006
8. Retardation	2.2	(1)	2.0	(1)	.05
9. Agitation	.31	(.6)	.41	(.6)	NS
10. Anxiety, psychic	2.2	(1)	2.3	(1.1)	NS
11. Anxiety, somatic	2.0	(1.2)	2.1	(1.1)	NS
12. Gastrointestinal	1.1	(.7)	1.1	(.7)	NS
13. General somatic	1.1	(.6)	1.1	(.6)	NS
14. Genital	1.7	(1.2)	1.2	(1.2)	.001
15. Hypochondriasis	1.6	(1.1)	1.7	(1.1)	NS
16. Loss of weight	.96	(.7)	.89	(.8)	NS
17. Loss of insight	.43	(.6)	.32	(.5)	NS

[a] Mean (SD)

Table 3. Dysthymia. Differences in HAM-D ratings according to sex ($n=774$)

	Male n=314		Female n=460		Two-tailed t-test
1. Depressed mood	2.2	(.8) [a]	2.2	(.8)	NS
2. Guilt	.94	(.9)	.91	(.9)	NS
3. Suicide	.61	(.7)	.61	(.7)	NS
4. Insomnia, initial	1.2	(.7)	1.34	(.7)	.05
5. Insomnia, middle	.68	(.6)	.71	(.6)	NS
6. Insomnia, delayed	.64	(.7)	.68	(.7)	NS
7. Work and interest	2.3	(1)	2.2	(.9)	.05
8. Retardation	1.2	(1)	1.1	(1)	NS
9. Agitation	1.36	(5)	1.4	(5)	NS
10. Anxiety, psychic	1.9	(.9)	2.0	(.9)	NS
11. Anxiety, somatic	1.9	(1)	2.1	(1)	NS
12. Gastrointestinal	.88	(.6)	.93	(.7)	NS
13. General somatic	1.13	(.6)	1.14	(.6)	NS
14. Genital	1.2	(1)	1.0	(1)	.05
15. Hypochondriasis	1.6	(.9)	1.4	(.9)	NS
16. Loss of weight	.58	(.7)	.71	(.7)	.05
17. Loss of insight	.45	(.5)	.44	(.5)	NS

[a] Mean (SD)

Table 4. Major depression (MD) and dysthymia (DD). Differences in HAM-D rating (n=1204)

	DD (n=774)		MD (n=430)		Two-tailed t-test
1. Depressed mood	2.3	(.8)[a]	3.1	(.9)	.001
2. Guilt	.9	(.9)	1.6	(.1)	.001
3. Suicide	.6	(.8)	1.2	(.1)	.001
4. Insomnia, initial	1.3	(.8)	1.3	(.8)	NS
5. Insomnia, middle	.7	(.7)	.9	(.7)	.001
6. Insomnia, delayed	.7	(.7)	1.2	(.8)	.001
7. Work and interest	2.2	(1)	2.9	(1)	.001
8. Retardation	1.2	(1)	2.1	(1)	.001
9. Agitation	.3	(.6)	.3	(.7)	NS
10. Anxiety, psychic	2.0	(1)	2.3	(1)	.001
11. Anxiety, somatic	2.0	(1)	2.1	(1)	NS
12. Gastrointestinal	.9	(.7)	1.6	(.7)	.001
13. General somatic	1.1	(.6)	1.2	(.6)	NS
14. Genital	1.1	(1)	1.5	(1)	.001
15. Hypochondriasis	1.5	(.9)	1.7	(1)	.01
16. Loss of weight	.7	(.7)	.9	(.8)	.01
17. Loss of insight	.45	(.5)	.37	(.6)	.02

[a] Mean (SD)

4.2 DSM-III Diagnoses and the HAM-D Scale

Table 2 shows the 430 cases with major depression and compares males and females. Three items differentiate the two subgroups: suicidal ideas (more common in females), impairment of work and interest (more common in males), and loss of libido (more common in males). Baumann (1976) in a German sample and Hamilton (1989) in a posthumous paper also found a difference in reported loss of libido; the latter however discounted this as an artefact. Hamilton (1989) also found that loss of energy was worse in females. This was not confirmed by our Spanish data.

The same analysis was carried out with the dysthymic sample (Table 3). This time four differences between the genders were found: initial insomnia, impairment of work and interest and loss of libido were more frequent among the males; loss of weight was more common among the females.

Table 4 shows that dysthymia and major depression differ in *all* but four items: initial insomnia, agitation, somatic anxiety and general somatic. This is of some interest as some of these symptoms used to be considered as characteristic of the old notion of neurotic depression that the category dysthymia has attempted to replace.

4.3 Item Analysis

Table 5 shows item/global score correlations. The first column includes data on dysthymia, the second on major depression, and the third on the total sample. Coefficients are higher for the major depression sample. This may simply

Table 5. Hamilton depression scale: Corrected item/global score correlations

	DD (n=774)	MD (n=430)	TS (n=1204)	C1[a] (n=141) (F)	C2[b] (n=213) (M)
1. Depressed mood	.32	.37	.46	.63	.76
2. Guilt	.24	.38	.39	.26	.39
3. Suicide	.26	.40	.39	.47	.44
4. Insomnia, initial	.25	.23	.25	.40	.49
5. Insomnia, middle	.32	.37	.37	.41	.55
6. Insomnia, delayed	.31	.42	.43	.37	.49
7. Work and interest	.39	.33	.46	.46	.60
8. Retardation	.24	.31	.34	.14	.46
9. Agitation	.24	.35	.22	.18	.57
10. Anxiety, psychic	.42	.36	.43	.54	.55
11. Anxiety, somatic	.35	.29	.33	.46	.54
12. Gastrointestinal	.33	.37	.39	.27	.55
13. General somatic	.29	.34	.32	.38	.50
14. Genital	.29	.30	.33	.13	.52
15. Hypochondriasis	.34	.36	.36	.33	.31
16. Loss of weight	.29	.26	.32	.25	.55
17. Loss of insight	.06	.06	−.00	.16	.41
Cronbach Alpha (Standardized)	.70	.74	.76	.76	?

[a] Rehm and O'Hara (1985)
[b] Mowbray (1972)
DD, dysthymia; MD, major depression; TS, total sample; C1, British sample; C2, American sample; (F), females only; (M), males only

reflect a wider range of scores or an intrinsic property of the scale which was, after all, designed to measure major depression. Coefficients for a British (Mowbray 1972) and an American sample (Rehm and O'Hara 1985) were not significantly higher than those for the Spanish sample. Table 5 also includes Alpha Cronbach values (Cronbach et al. 1972). The dysthymic group had the lowest coefficient. The Cronbach for the total Spanish sample is the same as that reported by Rehm and O'Hara (1985).

4.4 Factorial Structure

There has been great disparity in the number of factors reported in the literature. Table 6 shows the main studies. Discrepancies can be explained in various ways:

1. Scales with different numbers of items have been analysed. Attempts at improving the original scale have led to versions of up to 28 items. Analysis of these is likely to yield different factor structures.
2. Different extraction techniques have been used.
3. Different rotational methods have been used. Occasionally, unrotated factors have been reported. In general, there has been a preference for orthogonal rotations.

Table 6. Main factor analytic studies using the HAM-D scale

Author(s)	Number	Males/ females	Mean age (years)	Mean score	Items	Method	Rotation	Factors (interpreted)
Hamilton (1960)	49 [a]		?	?	17	FA	Varimax	4
Hamilton (1967a)	272	152/120	?	?	17	PCA	Varimax	6
Michaux et al. (1969)	158	54/104	35	?	17	FA	Varimax	7
Paykel et al. (1970)	220	57/163	?	?	28	PCA	No rotat.	3
Weckowicz et al. (1971)	52 [a]		?	?	17	PCA	Varimax	6
Mowbray (1972)	347	134/213	?	19	17	PCA	No rotat.	6
Sarteschi et al. (1973)	497	71/426	53	?	17	FA	Varimax	3
Cleary and Guy (1977)	779	312/467	38	?	23	PCA	Varimax	6
Guelfi et al. (1981)	272	152/120	?	?	26	PCA	Varimax	6
Dreyfus et al. (1981)	85	? ?	?		17	PCA	Varimax	4
Rhoades and Overall (1983)	420	? ?	?		21	FA	Oblique	7
Maier et al. (1985)	293	91/202	41	22	17/21	FA	Varimax	4
Cordero and Ramos (1986)	115	? ?	?		17	PCA	Varimax	5
O'Brien and Glaudin (1988)	365	256/109	35	22	17	PCA	Varimax	6
Berrios and Bulbena (1989)	1204	491/713	42	22	17	methods	Various	4

[a] Males only

4. Patient samples vary a great deal in terms of diagnosis and size. This raises the important statistical issue of the generalizability of the factor structures found.
5. The scale itself may have no structural invariance. However, 1 to 4 above must be thoroughly investigated before this explanation is accepted.

Table 7 shows the HAM-D factor structure in the Spanish major depression subsample. Complying with the suggestions of Comrey (1973) and other factorists, the sample was randomly divided into two subgroups of 220 and 210 subjects respective for halves A and B. Each half was factor-analyzed independently. To allow comparison with the work of O'Brien and Glaudin (1988) principal component analysis and varimax rotation were used throughout. We are at present systematically comparing the efficiency and clinical plausibility of other extraction and rotating algorithms, but these data will be reported elsewhere (Berrios and Bulbena 1990).

Subsamples A and B yielded four factors; their respective loadings are shown in the first eight columns of Table 7. Decimal points and negative signs

Table 7. Major depression. HAM-D factor structures – comparison of sample halves and controls

	Half A (n=220)				Half B (n=210)				Control [a] (n=183)			
	A1	A2	A3	A4	B1	B2	B3	B4	C1	C2	C3	C4
1. Depressed mood	49	36	25	03	46	26	24	12	75	02	15	08[b]
2. Guilt	50	44	03	24	45	43	01	04	44	09	03	05
3. Suicide	47	00	01	34	50	03	34	31	58	18	29	00
4. Insomnia, initial	41	20	13	14	34	11	11	53	15	15	36	25
5. Insomnia, middle	52	07	37	00	56	05	03	46	06	05	01	81
6. Insomnia, delayed	59	05	30	10	63	15	00	00	06	10	21	76
7. Work and interest	36	47	32	26	40	43	06	42	41	44	15	10
8. Retardation	31	63	12	00	38	53	09	26	23	04	05	13
9. Agitation	47	23	01	39	39	49	15	03	16	04	13	10
10. Anxiety, psychic	53	25	39	08	48	17	59	04	41	53	07	12
11. Anxiety, somatic	47	51	20	02	52	27	54	05	06	76	23	01
12. Gastrointestinal	52	27	40	28	42	32	38	06	10	02	78	14
13. General somatic	40	37	15	32	46	39	06	25	19	77	09	03
14. Genital	33	07	28	67	45	08	12	55	46	05	34	39
15. Hypochondriasis	50	06	13	35	50	38	14	07	20	50	07	41
16. Loss of weight	35	04	53	20	45	03	46	07	07	03	81	03
17. Loss of insight	00	39	45	03	17	39	40	13	04	03	08	04

Statistics: A1 vs B1: $r = .85$; A2 vs B2: $r = .86$; A3 vs B3: $r = .67$; A4 vs B4: $r = .57$
A1 vs C1: $r = .16$; A2 vs C2: $r = .54$; A3 vs C3: $r = .47$; A4 vs C4: $r = .09$
B1 vs C1: $r = .03$; B2 vs C2: $r = .32$; A3 vs C3: $r = .49$; A4 vs C4: $r = .17$

(cut-off r for factor homology: $= > .80$)

[a] O'Brien and Glaudin (1988)
[b] Decimal points and negative signs have been omitted for convenience

have been removed for reasons of space. The factors extracted by O'Brien and Glaudin (1988) from a sample of 183 subjects are shown in the last four columns.

Although subsamples A, B and that of O'Brien and Glaudin (1988) seem to have the same factorial structure, it is important to ascertain whether the four factors are homologous. One simple way to demonstrate homology is to correlate the corresponding factors. By convention homology is accepted when r is = or > than 0.8. Table 7 shows that when subsamples A and B were compared only the first two factors showed adequate homology. The lack of homology for factors 3 and 4 may reflect either the oversensitivity of the extraction algorithm or, less likely, a structural flaw in the scale itself. In favour of the former is that our factor structure compares well with that reported by Cordero and Ramos (1986).

There was no factorial homology between the Spanish and O'Brien and Glaudin (1988) samples. This discrepancy needs explanation in view of the fact that both studies included DSM-III major depressions, and used the same factor analytic algorithms and statistical package. *One explanation* might be that a cultural factor is at play. In this regard differences have been reported between African and European samples (Binitie 1975). *Another* that principal component analysis is an unstable technique in that it is oversensitive to the scatter of scores (Tinsley and Tinsley 1987). To test each of these hypotheses we need to compare the "endorsement patterns" in both samples. *A third explanation* is that the scale itself does not possess a reliable factorial structure. It is too early to conclude that this is the case, particularly because O'Brien and Glaudin (1988) have shown homology across their four factors.

5 Conclusions

The following conclusions can be drawn:

1. Further research into the Hamilton scale must take into consideration Hamilton's epistemological views and his theoretical preferences for scale construction.
2. Before any attempt is made to modify the scale, its structural characteristics and limits of applicability must be found.
3. Techniques have become available to do this work. Reports must try to uniformize their approach. Re-evaluation of past work is made difficult by the lack of uniformity and of information.
4. Factor analysis can be used with advantage, particularly since this technique has recovered from the bad press it once had. This should be supplemented by other statistical techniques (Bech et al. 1981).
5. Major depression and dysthymia showed significant endorsement pattern differences in the Spanish sample. A split-sample analysis of the major depression subsample showed homology only for the first two factors.
6. If done with statistical seriousness, this work would have satisfied Max Hamilton (1983) who recognized the preliminary nature of his scale: "I went around with my scale and it created a tremendous wave of apathy. They all thought I was a bit mad. Eventually it got published in the *Journal of Neurology, Neurosurgery and Psychiatry*. It was the only one that would take it. And now everyone tells me the scale is wonderful. I always remember when it had a different reception. This makes sure I don't get a swollen head" (p.63).

References

APA (1980) Diagnostic and statistical manual of mental disorders, 3rd edn American Psychiatric Association, Washington

Baumann U (1976) Methodische Untersuchungen zur Hamilton-Depression-Skala. Arch Psychiatr Nervenkr 222:359–375

Bech P (1981) Rating scales for affective disorders: their validity and consistency. Acta Psychiatr Scand [Suppl] 295:18–31

Bech P, Gram LF, Dein E, Jacobsen J, Vitger J, Bolwig T G (1975) Quantitative rating of depressive states. Acta Psychiatr Scand 51:161–170

Bech P, Bolwig TG, Kramp P, Rafaelsen OJ (1979) The Bech-Rafaelsen mania scale and the Hamilton depression scale. Evaluation of homogeneity and inter-observer reliability. Acta Psychiatr Scand 59:420–430

Bech P, Allerup P, Gram LF, Reisby N, et al. (1981) The Hamilton depressive scale. Evaluation of objectivity using logistic models. Acta Psychiatr Scand 63:290–299

Berrios GE (1984) Descriptive psychopathology: conceptual and historical aspects. Psychol Med 14:303–313

Berrios GE, Bulbena A (1990) Factorial structure of Hamilton depression scale and Dysthymia (in preparation)

Binitie A (1975) A factor-analytical study of depression across cultures (African and European). Br J Psychiatry 127:559–563

Brown W, Thomson GH (1925) The essentials of mental measurement. Cambridge University Press, Cambridge

Burt C (1940) The factors of the mind. University of London Press, London

Cleary P, Guy W (1977) Factor analysis of the Hamilton depression scale. Drugs Exp Clin Res 1:115–120

Comrey AL (1973) A first course in factor analysis. Academic, New York

Cordero Villafáfila A, Ramos-Brieva JA (1986) Estructura factorial de la versión castellana de la escala de Hamilton para la depresión. Actas Luso Esp Neurol Psiquiatr 14:339–342

Cronbach LJ, Gleser GC, Nanda H, Rajaratnam N (1972) The dependability of behavioral measurements. Wiley, New York

Dening TR, Berrios GE (1989) Wilson's disease: clinical groups in 400 cases. Acta Neurol Scand 80:527–534

Dreyfus JF, Guelfi JD, Ruschel C, Blanchard C, Pichot P (1981) Structure factorielle de l'échelle de dépression de Hamilton II. Ann Med Psychol (Paris) 139:446–453

Ghiselli EE, Campbell JP, Zedeck S (1981) Measurement theory for the behavioral sciences. Freeman, San Francisco

Guelfi JD, Dreyfus JF, Ruschel S, Blanchard C, Pichot P (1981) Structure factorielle de l'échelle de dépression de Hamilton I. Ann Med Psychol (Pans) 139:199–214

Fodor JA (1983) The modularity of mind. MIT Press, Cambridge

Hamilton M (1959) The assessment of anxiety states by rating. 5 Med Psychol 32:50–55

Hamilton M (1960) A rating scale for depression. J Neurol Neurosurg Psychiatry 26:56–62

Hamilton M (1965) Prediction in practice. In: Banks C, Bradhurst PL (eds) Studies in psychology. University of London Press, London, pp 109–118

Hamilton M (1967a) Development of a rating scale for primary depressive illness. Br J Soc Clin Psychol 6:278–296

Hamilton M (1967b) Comparison of factors by Ahmavaara's method. Br J Math Stat Psychol 20:107–110

Hamilton M (1983) In conversation with Max Hamilton. Bull R Coll Psychiatr 7:62–66

Hamilton M (1989) Frequency of symptoms in melancholia (depressive illness). Br J Psychiatry 154:201–206

Hearnshaw LS (1979) Cyril Burt. Psychologist. Hodder and Stoughton, London

Hedlund JL, Vieweg BW (1979) The Hamilton rating scale for depression: a comprehensive review. J Operat Psychiatry 10:149–162

Kim JO, Mueller CW (1978a) Introduction to factor analysis. Sage, London

Kim JO, Mueller CW (1978b) Factor analysis. Statistical methods and practical issues. Sage, London

Lawley DN, Maxwell AE (1963) Factor analysis as a statistical method. Butterworth, London

Maier W, Philipp M, Gerken A (1985) Dimensionen der Hamilton-Depressions-skala (HAMD). Eur Arch Psychiatry Neurol Sci 234:417–422

Michaux ME, Suziedelis A, Germize K, Rossi JA (1969) Depression factors in depressed and in heterogeneous in-patient samples. J Neurol Neurosurg Psychiatry 32:609–613

Mowbray RM (1972) The Hamilton rating scale for depression: a factor analysis. Psychol Med 2:272–280

O'Brien KP, Glaudin V (1988) Factorial structure and factor reliability of the Hamilton rating scale for depression. Acta Psychiatr Scand 78:113–120

Osterlind SJ (1983) Test item bias. Sage, London

Paykel ES, Norton KRW (1986) Self-report and clinical interview in the assessment of depression. In: Sartorius N, Ban TA (eds) Assessment of depression. Springer, Berlin Heidelberg New York, pp 356–366

Paykel ES, Klerman GL, Prussoff BA (1970) Treatment setting and clinical depression. Arch Gen Psychiatry 22:11–21

Politynska B, Berrios GE, Miller E (1990) The relationship between motor, depressive and cognitive symptoms in Parkinson's disease: a pattern recognition analysis. Behav Neurol (in press)

Ramos-Brieva JA, Cordero Villafáfila A (1986a) Validación de la versión castellana de la escala de Hamilton para la depresión. Actas Luso Esp Neurol Psquiatr 14:324–334

Ramos-Brieva JA, Cordero Villafáfila A (1986b) Relación entre validez y seguridad de la versión castellana de la escala de Hamilton para la depresión. Actas Luso Esp Neurol Psiquiatr 14:335–338

Ramos-Brieva JA, Cordero Villafáfila A (1987a) Características individuales de cada item de la escala de Hamilton para la depresión. Actas Luso Esp Neurol Psiquiatr 15:215–221

Ramos-Brieva JA, Cordero Villafáfila A (1987b) La escala de Hamilton para la depresión: versión breve de Bech o versión completa. Actas Luso Esp Neurol Psiquiatr 15:209–214

Rehm LP, O'Hara MW (1985) Item characteristics of the Hamilton rating scale for depression. J Psychiatr Res 19:31–41

Rhoades HM, Overall JE (1983) The Hamilton Depression scale: factor analysis scoring and profile classification. Psychopharmacol Bull 19:91–96

Robins LN (1989) Diagnostic grammar and assessment: translating criteria into questionnaires. Psychol Med 19:57–68

Sarteschi P, Cassano GB, Castrogiovanni P, Conti L (1973) The use of rating scales for computer analysis of the affective symptoms in old age. Compr Psychiatry 14:371–379

Shallice T (1988) From neuropsychology to mental structure. Cambridge University Press, Cambridge

Spearman C (1932) The abilities of man. Macmillan, London

Thomson G (1950) The factorial analysis of human ability. University of London Press, London

Thurstone LL (1947) Multiple-factor analysis. University of Chicago Press, Chicago

Tinsley HEA, Tinsley DJ (1987) Uses of factor analysis in counseling psychology research. J Counsel Psychol 34:414–424

Weckowicz TE, Cropley AJ, Muir W (1971) An attempt to replicate the results of a factor analytic study in depressed patients. J Clin Psychol 27:30–31

Ziegler VE, Meyer DA, Rosen SH, Biggs JT (1978) Reliability of video-taped Hamilton ratings. Biol Psychiatry 13:119–122

Subject Index